June,
With love and a[...]
for your devotion & service
to our Lord Jesus Christ

Love
Roy Phil 1:6; 2:13

God

and the

Sexual Metaphor

Theological Implications and Behavioral Guidelines

Roy C. Price
DMin, DPhil

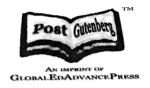

AN IMPRINT OF
GLOBALEDADVANCEPRESS

God and the Sexual Metaphor

Theological Implications and Behavioral Guidelines

Copyright © 2015 Roy C. Price

Library of Congress Control Number: 2015942876

Price, Roy Cantrell   1935 -

God and the Sexual Metaphor

ISBN 978-1-935434-77-1

Subject Codes and Description: 1. HEA042000: Health and Fitness: Sexuality
2. REL012050: Religion: Christian Life – Love and Marriage
3. REL067000: Religion: Theology - General

Cover design by Brian Lane Green

Printed in Australia, Brazil, France, Germany, Italy, Poland, Russia, Spain, UK,
USA, and wherever there is an Espresso Book Machine

The Press does not have ownership of the contents of a book; this is the
author's work and the author owns the copyright. All theory,
concepts, constructs, and perspectives are those of the author and not
necessarily the Press. They are presented for open and free discussion
of the issues involved. All comments and feedback should be directed
to the Email: [comments4author@aol.com] and the comments will be
forwarded to the author for response.

Order books from www.gea-books.com/bookstore/
or any place good books are sold.

Published by
Post-Gutenberg Books
An Imprint of
GlobalEdAdvancePRESS

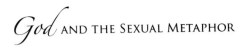

CONTENTS

Publisher's Preface

God and the Sexual Metaphor clarifies sexual activity and behavioral guidelines found in sacred writings. The purpose is to define the sexual metaphor used by God to describe His relationship with His people, and thereby understanding the boundaries established in Scripture for sensual expression.

Dr. Roy Price, a knowledgeable Christian leader, discusses the essential sacred concepts in an effort to assist parents, pastors, and youth to have a more compelling argument for sexual activity within the boundary of marriage and against sex as a sport. Using the Word of God as a guide to human behavior, the author discusses the benefits of following moral guidelines and the consequences for contrary behavior. Dr. Price asserts that God's plan is good and that the consequences are marked with impartiality.

Dr. Price writes on the assumption that God designed sex, not man or society, and that human sexual expression in the context of marriage is good in the sight of God. He further believes the Bible is a guide to human behavior which includes sexual expression. Dr. Price also states that there are benefits in conforming to God's guidelines and consequences when one does not conform. He believes human beings are born in a sinful condition that causes an inwardly desire to do the opposite of God's will. He affirms that this condition can be changed by a relationship with Jesus Christ. Pastors, parents, youth and youth workers can benefit from the study of this work, which is an extension of a pastor's heart.

— **Hollis L Green, ThD, PhD, DLitt**

Roy Price's manuscript about 'God and the Sexual Metaphor' is fascinating. It is such a delight to read something positive about the idea of sex from an evangelical. Roy is accurate in handling the text of Scripture, and he is oh so practical. I would love to listen to multiple Bible teachers interact with this manuscript and the text of Scripture. While outside the scope of this manuscript's emphasis, I would love to see Dr. Price write a sequel addressing the concept of marriage and its vows with the same focus and intensity as this volume.

— Patrick A. Blewett, DMin, PhD
Dean of A.W. Tozer Theological Seminary

Our living in Christ is a deep intimacy God desires to have with those who belong to Him. Dr. Roy Price has labored intensely over many years to build his understanding of what the incarnation, indwelling, and inhabiting of Christ . . . God Himself living within us . . . mean in human experience. This volume will help the reader grow in this understanding so that this deep, passionate experience of intimacy with God can be both more fully understood and more intentionally nurtured.

— Dr. Bob Fetherlin
President, One Mission Society

Dr. Roy Price has written a timely book that brings a Judeo-Christian biblical worldview to the issues of human sexuality. The contemporary culture is saturated with images and models of sexual behavior, and we constantly receive advice about how we should behave as sexual beings. Price's book is a breath of clean air. It deserves a wide audience.

— Lyle W. Dorsett, PhD
Billy Graham Professor of Evangelism,
Beeson Divinity School

FOREWORD

Of all the complexities of the human organism the sexual instinct fusion is undoubtedly the apogee. Civilization has looked at sexual activities and practices in divergent ways from the narcissism of passion, to the rationalization of worship, to the ultimate in agape.

Even in the Evangelical community the perception of sexual activity has changed. It is not so many years ago that sexual activity was considered exclusively the mechanism of producing children and heirs. Even the very thought that there might be something physically enjoyable in the act of intimacy was abhorrent and often considered sinful in itself. Today we have arrived at the far end of the morality spectrum in which sex outside of marriage is considered normal and those who do not accept this view are old-fashioned.

Why is it then that God chose sexual intimacy as a metaphor to communicate His closeness to His people? Surely another method with less emotional charge might have been easier for everyone.

What is the experience in sexual intimacy?

First, it may be a manifestation of a purely narcissistic enterprise in which the partner is of no personal importance or significance and is the mere mechanical apparatus to ensure personal satisfaction and relief.

Secondly, it may be the ultimate expression and experience of agape – the antithesis of narcissism – in which the desire of both participants is for the satisfaction, pleasure and fulfillment of the other. In such a state the self is absorbed into the person of the partner and psychologically for a period of time both become one.

We should not be surprised, therefore, to discover that as the world degenerates into the narcissistic slough of selfishness – politically, economically and ecclesiastically - that intimacy has degenerated into selfism.

God in His wisdom selected the sexual encounter as the concrete and personal representation of the special relationship between Himself and His children. The ultimate measurement of spiritual maturity is the legal standard, 'What is in the best interest of God,' and the enfolding of oneself within the personality of God. This is His desire. As biological sex is a recrudescence of an attempt to reenter the security of the mother's womb so is the spiritual experience of the new birth depicted by the biological experience.

This is a book that should have been written fifty years ago for the benefit of the evangelical community. We are all in debt to Dr. Price for teaching us about a most important subject that so often is the concern of hedonism, and elevating our perspective above the standard of the secular world to not only having a fulfilled marriage relationship but to an intimacy with God - an elevation that comes not from Freud but exclusively from the energizing power of God's spirit.

—**E. Basil Jackson, MD, PhD, JD**
Distinguished Professor of Psychiatry, Medicine, And Law

INTRODUCTION

It has been my privilege to serve in various aspects of evangelical pastoral ministries in various sections of the United States for over fifty-five years. I began as a club director in Youth for Christ, served in smaller rural and suburban churches, inner city, the International Church in Saigon, Vietnam at the end of U. S. involvement, and led multiple staffs in larger churches in northern California. My wife and I have enjoyed almost fifty-eight years of marriage at this writing. We met in college and each of us was a virgin when we married. Our marriage has been in the norm of experience as two very differently wired people have sought to live together to enjoy one another, honor and serve God.

During the last half-century it is obvious that approaches by society and the Christian church to promiscuous sex have had little impact on youth or adult behavior. There is an abundance of books on the psychological aspects of sexual relations and an exhaustless list on how to have great sex as though an orgasm is the answer to all of life. One actress said we are in an orgasmic culture. Narcissism and hedonistic pursuit of pleasure as the highest good dominate the entertainment industry. The sexual revolution of the sixties with the advent of the pill and widespread use of drugs escalated promiscuity. Previously accepted traditional concepts of sex within the boundary of marriage were replaced by a relaxed attitude toward morality in which 'how can something that feels so good be wrong'. It flourished in the fertile seedbed of moral relativism. Nothing is new about sex; it is as old as the Garden of Eden. Go Daddy, Hooters and Carl's Jr. know how to arouse the male with voluptuous, seductive models.

When AIDS broke on the scene in the eighties, some thought there would follow a pullback in promiscuous sex. It became only a short pause. More explicit sex on television and the explosion of pornography on the Internet have merged to amplify sex to a near religious level in a search for meaning and fulfillment.

Over twenty-five years ago while engaged in my annual read-the-Bible through, I was struck by the frequent references to God accusing Israel and Judah of adulterous behavior. I asked the question, why did God use the sexual metaphor to describe His relationship to His people, Israel and Judah? He did not choose lying (the tongue), theft or the violence of murder, but the most private, personal activity of humanity as the metaphor of choice. What does this tell us about sex and about God? Is there something in sex, which God created, that elevates it above all other behavior and puts it in a separate category? If sex can be seen through a theological lens, will it be a helpful tool for pastors, teachers, and parents to help their students establish boundaries and empower them to say 'No' to sexual advances and normal sex drives until fulfilled in marriage? Will this enable adults in marriage or single life to avoid increased disappointment and heartache sex outside of marriage usually brings?

The purpose of the book is to define the metaphor of sex used by God to describe His relationship to His people, and thereby understand the reasons for the boundaries established in the Bible for the expression of sexual behavior. The book begins with references to a couple of movies that reflected the negative side of promiscuity. I propose that the Bible's view of sex is not irrelevant or outdated in a supposedly sophisticated culture. To support my contentions I explore the use of metaphor and the theological underpinnings of the sexual metaphor. I argue that the metaphor demands personal integrity for sexual relationships to bring the intimacy and fulfillment people desire. Integrity, in turn, directs us to the character of God and the relationship of the Trinity. The challenge of my attempt is whether or not this elevation of sex to the highest category of Triune relationships will be strong enough to help youth and adults realize the power and beauty found in God's parameters for sexual fulfillment.

What every person, believer and unbeliever alike, faces is the internal conflict of a dynamic drive that wants sex immediately and the voices of conscience, personal standards or family culture that push for restraint. This battle is weighted in favor of indulgence by the prevalence of a media that has few boundaries and those that it has are very porous. In biblical terms for the Christian, it is described as a flesh/Spirit push-pull conflict. Does the God who established the boundaries also provide a solution to the problem of sexual restraint? The internal power to keep within the boundaries is found in personal regeneration and the empowering of the Holy Spirit in the individual. To help the reader, I provide a Bible study based on 2 Peter 1:3-11 and the seven character qualities the believer is to develop.

Benefits of following God's plan include the satisfaction of a life-long relationship, increased personal worth and personal security. The consequence of choosing to disregard the boundaries is the reality of judgment by a good and just God. Humanity is free to choose behaviors, but not free to determine the consequences of their choices.

My experience has been that Christian leaders' knee-jerk response to a problem is to write a rule of prohibition to attempt to control behavior and produce spiritual life. I go back to the rules of early church councils to demonstrate this approach has never worked. The moral failure of leaders within the Christian church strongly demonstrates that it takes more than merely establishing a 'don't-have-sex-outside of a man-woman marital relationship'. The struggle of Christian leaders to cope with the power of the sex-drive goes back to the early centuries of Christianity. Seeking to control sex by ecclesiastical law demonstrably failed. Something must happen to change the heart of the human and provide divine power to stay within God's boundaries. That something is the good news, the Gospel of a living Savior Who changes the heart by the personal presence of the Holy Spirit. A life pleasing to God that leads to personal joy and peace is possible through Christ, through whom we can live within God's parameters.

A summary of assumptions in my approach to this subject:

1. The Bible is the inerrant Word of God and therefore an infallible guide to human behavior and sexual expression.

2. There are benefits for conforming to God's guidelines, and consequences for not conforming; in both cases, God acts justly and wisely. Just means God's established consequences are fair and wise means His plan is for the good and blessing of all people.

3. All humanity is born disadvantaged with the handicap of sin, a condition that causes a person to inwardly desire to do the opposite of God's will. It is only through the saving grace of God in Jesus Christ that the heart can be changed, and by the dynamic of the Holy Spirit that behavior can be conformed to the will of a holy God.

4. If an idea is important enough and compelling, it can control the strongest passions of the human body and personality. It is my hope that by discussing this fundamental biblical concept, parents, youth and pastors will have a more compelling argument against sex as a sport and for sex within the boundary of the marriage of a man and woman.

5. At best, people understand and behave with limited perfection.

I have capitalized the personal pronoun in reference to deity except in quotations where the author did not do so or in biblical quotes where translators did not so capitalize. The New International Bible is used unless otherwise designated.

1

IS SEX SOUL-DESTROYING OR SOUL-FULFILLING?

The first two things we learn about sex from God, right from the beginning, are that God designed it, not man or society, and that it is very good. (Peter Kreeft)[1]

"Are Jay and Claire in love? The script suggests not, indicating that sorrow and need—not passion—have brought these adulterers together. (Jay has a wife and two young sons at home.) What's more, the movie makes plain, physical intimacy need not lead to emotional intimacy. For all they have shared, Jay and Claire remain strangers to one another, their couplings clinical and willfully anonymous and—on some level—soul-destroying." So wrote one review of the 2001 film 'Intimacy.' The film is based on a book with the same title by Hanif Kureishi. 'Intimacy' is a movie in which a man and a woman meet for short, brutal, anonymous sex every Wednesday afternoon. They want to keep it to that: no names, no small talk, wrote Roger Ebert[2]. As Ebert continued his review, he

---

1   Peter Kreeft, http://www.peterkreeft.com/topics-more/sexual-symbolism.htm
2   http://www.rogerebert.com/reviews/intimacy-2001

suggested the male was really looking for something more than raw sex.

Can sex be soul-destroying? Most of the media, from rap to pop to film and video argue the opposite. However, this movie addresses this soul-destroying potential, refuting the false, yet popular claim that the person who has the most sex with the most people—like celebrity athletes or the exploits of political or entertainment figures—has the happiest, most fulfilling life. Is sex no more than unbridled, animal passion? Have the novelists, movie moguls, rappers, talk shows and soaps been selling us a dish of poison presented as a succulent filet mignon?

What can be wrong with something that feels so good, asked the once popular song. "I'm a 16-year-old Christian who recently gave up my virginity. I waited until I really loved my boyfriend, and I knew he loved me. I don't think sex has anything to do with the fact that you're married or single. I think it's a choice each person has to make by asking themselves if they're prepared for the outcome if something goes wrong. I talked to my partner about the possible outcomes. We used protection and nothing bad happened."[3] Does that sound like a pretty good argument to you? Is that how your peers view sex? Might there be some consequences that haven't been looked at other than pregnancy and STD's, or worse, AIDS?

This is a popular if not prevalent view of sex today. Our culture has defaulted to 'hook-ups'. There is a preponderance

3   ChristianityToday.com, Teens - "Love, Sex & Real Life," emails to Tim Stafford, © 2001 by the author or Christianity Today International/Campus Life magazine

of 'I think' in this statement justifying sexual choices. This girl concluded that it was her prerogative to evaluate the messages received from family and culture and then form a worldview—a view of how things work. Her view was that if you protect yourself from pregnancy and disease, sex is for feeling good. She failed to 'think' that there are other perspectives of sex than orgasm. She failed to 'think' of sex in spiritual and psychological terms. She failed to 'think' in long-term, whole-life terms. She failed to take into her thinking that sex is not an isolated physical act that brings a high level of sensual thrill. It involves a person's soul and spirit. In fact, the spirit of a person is core to sexual experience. And the violation of the spirit results in psychological (or soul) ramifications that go very deep. She went on to say they had recently broken up—a clear admission that sex doesn't prove love nor does it bring true intimacy and a lasting relationship.

In 'Vanilla Sky,' Penelope Cruz explodes on Tom Cruise in a powerful scene. She is driving and shouting at her lover that when you sleep with somebody your body makes a commitment even if your mind doesn't. That is true, but why? With our obvious pre-occupation with sex, why aren't we the most fulfilled society of all history? Because the Person who created sex has been ignored, there is an all-out hedonistic determination to have as much sensual thrill as possible. Yet the results have been broken hearts, marriages, and families, children having babies, single-parent homes and hollow lives. T. S. Eliot penned contemporary humanity:

We are the hollow men
We are the stuffed men
Leaning together
Headpiece filled with straw. Alas!
Our dried voices, when
We whisper together
Are quiet and meaningless
As wind in dry grass
Or rats' feet over broken glass
In our dry cellar[4]

She was in her mid-thirties, shapely with dark flowing shoulder length hair. A full bosom lifted her clothing with sensual enticement. She had already gone through five marriages that began when she was sixteen. There was a deep-seated, unsatisfied longing for closeness, acceptance, intimacy. She knew sex had its highs but by now she knew there was something more, something missing. She had found a new lover yet the old longing persisted.

The women in the small town where she lived had isolated her as little more than a prostitute. The men who looked at her mentally undressed her and wondered if they might get some action with her.

This day was hot. Most of the women in town had chosen to stay in their homes so she went into town to get water and some fruit and vegetables. The city well was located in the town center. As she approached she encountered a man who asked if she would draw some water for him to have a drink.

The next few moments would change her life—forever.

---

4   T.S. Eliot, "The Hollow Men", *T..S. Eliot Collected Poems: 1909-1962* (New York: Harcourt, Brace, Brace & World, Inc. 1970), 79.

"Hold on," she replied. "You're asking me for a drink? You're of a different race and racial bigotry has prevented your people from even talking to my people for centuries."

He responded, "If you would ask me I will give you living water."

"What kind of come-on is this? Our fore-fathers dug this well by hand. It's over 100' deep. You don't even have a bucket or rope and you will give me water—living, fresh, running water?"

Knowing the woman was desperately thirsty in her soul and spirit, longing for the satisfaction of knowing God, Jesus replied: "Everyone who drinks this water will be thirsty again, but whoever drinks the water I give him will never thirst. Indeed, the water I give him will become in him a spring of water welling up to eternal life."

"Sir, give me this water so that I won't get thirsty...."[5]

A person's view of how things are put together and work is known as a worldview. Even when an individual has not articulated his or her worldview, he or she makes choices and does things in sync with that mindset. This is true with sex. How we view sex is much more than mere animal instinct. A person will seek a promiscuous life in harmony with a *Playboy* worldview that treats sex as a sport. That can be in a homo or hetero-sexual relationship. Or, a person will enjoy a full sexual life within the defined boundaries of male and female marriage in concert with how they understand life works.

---

5   Read the rest of the story and its conclusion in John 4. The biblical account is embellished by the author.

If this is on target, then the origin of sex becomes crucial. The root of recreational sex is the result of a view that human beings are the highest level of evolution and nothing more. Therefore, sexual impulses and drives are on the same level of the animal. Sex is just monkeying around and having fun. In contrast, if God is the Creator, then sex was made and given its qualities by Him. Since all He does is purposeful, then sex is purposeful. If sex has divine purpose, then our attempts to make it recreational are doomed to bring suffering and heartache, not fulfillment. What, then, is its purpose and how can we discover it?

I Dreamed a Dream[6]

There was a time when men were kind
When their voices were soft
And their words inviting
There was a time when love was blind
And the world was a song
And the song was exciting
There was a time
Then it all went wrong

I dreamed a dream in time gone by
When hope was high
And life worth living
I dreamed that love would never die
I dreamed that God would be forgiving

---

6   http://www.allmusicals.com/lyrics/lesmiserables/idreamedadream.htm (accessed March 12, 2015).

Then I was young and unafraid
So dreams were made and used and wasted
There was no ransom to be paid
No song unsung
No wine untasted

But the tigers come at night
With their voices soft as thunder
As they tear your hope apart
And they turn your dream to shame

He slept a summer by my side
He filled my days with endless wonder
He took my childhood in his stride
But he was gone when autumn came
And still I dream he'll come to me
That we will live the years together
But there are dreams that cannot be
And there are storms we cannot weather

I had a dream my life would be
So different from this hell I'm living
So different now from what it seemed
Now life has killed
The dream I dreamed

Sex can generate the worst of crimes of which humans are capable. Or, it can lift the soul to transcendent power and beauty. It is godlike in goodness and beauty, or it can degenerate into evil and hideousness.

2

GETTING A DIFFERENT PERSPECTIVE

At the end of the Second World War, there was a significant change in the predominant aim of secular intellectuals, a shift of emphasis from utopianism to hedonism. The shift began slowly at first, then gathered speed. (Paul Johnson)[7]

There isn't anything 'wrong' with sex *per se*. However, when appropriate boundaries are discarded a lot goes wrong. It can be 'soul-destroying' and evidently there are some in our orgasmic culture that are beginning to understand this. In these pages we will seek to explore some of the spiritual roots of sex as expressed in the Bible. In doing so it is hoped that the reader will be convinced that the beauty, power and fulfillment the Creator intended for sexual experience is a good thing and will make choices appropriate to that view.

The Bible affirms that sex is good. God made it and said it was good. He also affirmed that the marriage bed is pure (Hebrews 13:4). Sex is not only good, it is one of the most

---

7   Paul Johnson, *The Intellectuals (New York: Harper & Row, Publishers, 1988),306.*

wonderful experiences God has given to humanity. And it isn't just for procreation, either. Sex is fun. It is powerful. It can absorb a person's whole interest if he or she lets it and so become addictive and distorted. Perverted sexual drive has caused some of the most horrific crimes in history. Peter Kreeft wrote: "If everything in nature means something, then the big things in nature mean something big. And sex is a Big Thing. What it means is so big that we will never exhaust it, only discover more facets of its diamond. But it is there, a massive fact of nature, not a clever human idea."[8]
Let's look at the bigness of sex.

Sex is designed to bring fulfillment in the welding of a husband and wife, the satisfaction of acceptance, and the affirmation of security and permanence. It was designed by its Creator to reflect His love and integrity. Philip Yancey described it: "The very word sex comes from a Latin verb that means to cut off or sever, and sexual impulses drive us to unite to restore somehow the union that has been severed. Freud diagnosed the deep pain within as a longing for union with a parent; Jung diagnosed a longing for union with the opposite sex. The Christian sees a deeper longing, for union with the God who created us. Sex prefigures that union by bringing together body and soul in a kind of wholeness not otherwise known."[9]

---

8   Peter Kreeft, http://www.peterkreeft.com/topics-more/sexual-symbolism.htm, (accessed 4/15/08, page 1)
9   Philip Yancey, *Designer Sex* (InterVarsity Press, Taken from *Rumors of Another World* by Philip D. Yancey. Copyright © 2003 by SCCI. Used by permission of The Zondervan Corporation), 5.

Sex is religious, not just physical. Sex and God are inextricably bound together. 'Good sex' is an expression and gift of a good God. Sex becomes evil when it is diverted from its purpose. God made sex as one dimension of all of nature in general and in the human species in particular. He made it so powerful that it insured the continuation of the species. He also endowed it with such beauty that he used it to describe the intimacy of His relationship to His people. Sex is a dominant drive in a healthy person. However, when sex controls a person it can lead to addictive and perverted behaviors that result in spiritual and psychological emptiness. Sex can generate the worst of crimes of which humans are capable. Or, it can lift the soul to transcendent power and beauty. It is godlike in goodness and beauty, or it can degenerate into evil and hideousness.

Tim Stafford penned a response to the question raised by the sixteen-year-old cited earlier in which he contrasted an 'individualistic' view of sex that brings two people together to enjoy the moment with a Christian view of a permanent relationship. In the latter, the enjoyment is present, not for a moment but a lifetime. He concluded: "You meet someone, decide to have sex, then go your separate ways. As long as you used protection, 'nothing bad happened.' But I'd say that something bad did happen to you and your boyfriend. A bond that was meant to be permanent was treated like a throwaway. People who love each other enough to expose their bodies and their love to each other in total vulnerability aren't meant to ever be torn apart. Even though you don't regret anything, I'd be surprised if the memories of that first, failed relationship don't haunt you. Sex is not just a physical thing. It's spiritual. When you tear apart after sex, there are consequences. At the very least, this first relationship will make your next relationship more likely to fail, because you've laid down some tracks you'll tend to follow again."

A simple illustration will help drive Stafford's point. When tape is stuck to one surface and then pulled up and stuck to another and pulled up and so on, it gradually loses its ability to bond each time it is joined with a new surface. Sex bonds two people together and it was designed by the Originator to be a permanent bond. To play the tape trick ends up destroying the purpose. To 'stick' one's self to multiple partners tragically leads to destroying the hope of long-term meaningful bonding. Consequently, the lack of meaningful and long term bonding leads to addictive sexual patterns in an attempt to fill the deep longings for love and attachment. 'Good sex' is an expression and gift of a good God. Sex becomes evil when it is perverted from its purpose.

Now let's explore the purpose of sex. To do so we need to move Stafford's argument for relationship into the spiritual realm: God designed sex to illustrate His love for humanity. God created sex as a metaphor, a word picture, of His relationship with humanity, not only as a means to a wonderful human relationship. Sex reflects the integrity of God's commitment to humanity to love, cherish and provide for us. Every day—twenty-four/seven/three-sixty-five—God is actively loving, cherishing and providing for His creation. To enable us to understand the depth of His loving grace, He gave to us a picture so that we could understand His love. However, sin has blinded our spiritual eyes to see behind the physical and so grasp the core idea. As God declared, the consequence of sin is disintegration (2 Peter 1:4 JBP). We have the evidence in the brokenness of human relationships and personalities strewn across the parched wasteland of recreational sex. In contrast, is the evidence of a husband and wife that followed God's pattern of a welded relationship to love, cherish and provide for each other throughout their lives even as they struggle through the conflicts of married life. This brings us to the intent of this book.

Out of the many possible metaphors that God might have chosen to picture His commitment and integrity, He used sex because when he created it He designed it to bring a man and woman together in intensive bonding. The word the Bible uses to refer to the strength of that bond is 'weld' (Genesis 2:24 'united' קָבַּד *daw-bak'*). In this permanent relationship two people can be honest and vulnerable because they know it is secure and won't be stripped away from them. Without a strong bond, insecurity, defensiveness, protecting turf, and watching our back-side with suspicion, characterize a marriage.

To enable us to understand His relationship to us, God put it in terms of sex. Why? Because sex was specifically designed by Him to be an expression of trust; trust based upon integrity, so that the commitment to give one's body to another person is not trashed like used tissue. God doesn't use people and throw them away. His commitment caused Him to become a human being, suffer rejection, misunderstanding, and finally crucifixion from the explicit motivation of love. "I have loved

you with an everlasting love," He wrote in Jeremiah 31:3.
He doesn't want a fickle in-and-out relationship with us. He
wants us to commit in permanence to Him as He has to us.
Sex was designed to illustrate the profound, spiritual nature of
intimacy—the very thing Jay and Claire missed in their sexual
trysts as Matt Wolf so accurately points out in his Associated
Press Review.

Throughout the Old Testament, sexual references serve as
a metaphor of God's relationship to His people. God spoke
of 'knowing' certain people—the same language used of the
sexual act. The Hebrew for 'know' means 'to be intimately
involved with a person.'[10] In a different sexual idiom, He
said His people, Judah and Israel, were prostitutes and
adulterers when they worshipped the Canaanite gods. The
word *adultery* occurs in forty-five verses of the NIV Bible,
and prostitution and derivatives appear in 108 verses. This
indicates the importance of the subject with many of the
passages referring to the religious adultery or prostitution of
God's people. Why didn't God compare idolatry to violence,
thievery or even murder? Why did God choose the sexual
metaphor? An understanding of the theological background
of sex as expressed through this metaphor provides insights
into the rationale of the Scriptural restraints placed on sexual
expression and the serious consequences of disobedience. That,
in turn, gives another tool in confronting the promiscuous
philosophy that permeates culture today.

---

10   James I. Packer, Merrill C. Tenney, William White, Jr., eds., *The Bible
Almanac*, (Nashville, Thomas Nelson Publishers, 1980), 453

Ideas are powerful and direct human behavior. Paul Johnson (*Intellectuals*, 1988) wrote of the intellectuals whose ideas have shaped the twentieth and twenty-first centuries. His book was an exposé of their dysfunctional personal lives. Most of these powerful individuals were moral profligates who wrote imposing their moral concepts on the rest of the world, even though their lives were often out of control. It is evident that the church has not been able to convince its own constituents or the secular culture that the boundary of a heterosexual monogamous marriage is best for the individual and for society. One Protestant group blamed the sexual malaise on 'outmoded attitudes' or ideas in the church. Rather than holding to the biblical mandate for heterosexual, monogamous marriage, it called for 'just-love' and placed Scripture as a secondary authority. The problem is not the Bible's relevance. It might be more correctly understood as a failure to grasp the why of biblical mandates. Our culture may well be described as orgasmic-centrist where advertising and entertainment focuses on casual sexual experiences rather than on long-term, committed relationships within heterosexual, monogamous marriage, a value once held primary by western civilization. The titillating excitement of flirtatious encounters sells products and is portrayed as the ultimate adventure. Because it 'sells' doesn't mean it's the best or even good. The teen icons of entertainment are taking off more clothes and gyrating in sexual innuendo in ever-increasing suggestion.

What is a metaphor and how is it used in the Bible to uncover the meaning of sex?

S exuality is core to our personhood. It is far more than a conjugal act. God created us to enjoy an intimate, committed relationship to Him, which is demonstrated in the sexual relationship of a man and woman in a committed marital relationship.

3

THE SEXUAL METAPHOR

About Metaphors

Every good poet knows that natural symbols are like the essential structures of language itself, unchangeable. The sky is, always was, and always will be a natural symbol for heaven; dirt is not. The eye's seeing is a natural symbol for the mind's understanding; the gut's groaning is not. We all know and recognize this unconsciously…. Everything is connected, and everything points beyond itself—especially sex (Peter Kreeft).[11]

Why did God choose the sexual metaphor to describe His relationship to His people? It is a question that has challenged me for years. Sex is certainly the focus of many books and articles, but this narrow slice of our inquiry explores why the ancient Hebrew people are charged with spiritual adultery because of their worship of pagan fertility gods. The people sought to syncretize with the pagan culture God intended for them to replace. As a consequence, their understanding of sex degenerated into fertility religion where sex with priests or

---

11   Peter Kreeft, http://www.peterkreeft.com/topics-more/sexual-symbolism. htm, (accessed 4/15/08, pages 1,2

priestesses was a metaphor of crop and animal reproduction and therefore prosperity. However, the Hebrew people did not go as far as their neighbor cultures. Jones clarifies: "A major distinction between the Hebraic people and the pagan cultures about them was their refusal to overly spiritualize sex, by attributing genital sexuality to God, or to degrade the gift of sexuality in general by attributing its origins to Satan or the fall. While genital sexuality in marriage was affirmed in the Old Testament, harsh condemnation was expressed for extramarital genital sexuality."[12]

We learn by moving from what we know to what we do not know. A metaphor is a word picture of a concept. 'He is a rock' is a word picture of a man's character and stability. 'Her eyes are like the reflection of the azure sky on a quiet pond' is a simile. Abstract thought is best grasped through concrete illustrations. Tremper Longman III, described the role of the metaphor in *Song of Songs*: "Metaphor has long been considered the master image or even the essence of poetry by literary scholars since the time of Aristotle. Metaphor presents a stronger connection between the two objects of comparison and is truly figurative language.... Metaphor catches our attention by the disparity between the two objects and the daring suggestion of similarity. Readers must ponder and reflect on the point of the similarity and, by so doing explore multiple levels of meaning and experience the emotional overtones of the metaphor."[13]

---

12   Jones, 1065.
13   Tremper Longman III, *Song of Songs* (Grand Rapids, Michigan: William B. Eerdmans Publishing Co., 2001), 13.

In support of his assertion, Kreeft referred to C. S. Lewis: "One of the ends for which sex was created was to symbolize to us the hidden things of God. One of the functions of human marriage is to express the nature of the union between Christ and the Church."[14] My contention is that the metaphor transmits us into the core relationship of the Trinity. The argument is that if a person understands the true spiritual nature of sex, they will be more willing to respect and implement the disciplines of delayed gratification and confinement of sex to the covenanted marital relationship of a man and woman. I propose that ideas and understanding, especially of God's nature, are powerful enough to control the God-implanted drives and impulses that, undisciplined, lead to destruction and disintegration (2 Peter 1:3-4, JBP). With that foundation in place, a person will be more willing to follow the strategies Paul provided by crucifying the flesh (*sarx*), with its passions and lusts.

Theological Underpinnings of the Metaphor

The above are but a few of the abundant references to the association of religion with sex. I have provided a more exhaustive list in the Appendix. Why are there so many references? Theologically, it begins with the nature of the Trinity. *Perichorēsis* refers to the interpenetration of the Godhead, the existence of persons in one another. Although God is not sexual, an intimacy exists within the Godhead that human sexuality is designed to represent. We must recognize that God has expressed Himself, among other things, in

---

14   Kreeft, *Ibid.*

feminine terms. John Stott emphasized full weight must be given...

> to those passages of Scripture which speak of God in feminine—and especially maternal—terms. For these texts help to illumine the nature and quality of Yahweh was not only 'the Rock who fathered you' but also 'the God who gave you birth'. This is a remarkable statement that he was simultaneously Israel's Father and Mother. In consequence, Israel could be sure of God's preserving faithfulness. For though a human mother might 'forget the baby at her breast and have no compassion on the child she has borne', yet, Yahweh promised, 'I will not forget you!' Instead, he would unfailingly love and console his people: 'As a mother comforts her child, so will I comfort you'.... Then Jesus himself on occasion used feminine imagery, likening God to a woman who had lost a coin, as well as to a father who had lost a son, and likening himself in his anguish over impenitent Jerusalem to a hen wanting to gather her chicks under her wings.[15] (Deuteronomy 32:18, cf. Isaiah 42:14; 49:15; 66:13; Psalm 131:1ff; Luke 15:8ff; Matthew 23:37).

When God created humanity male and female, His intention was that a parenting relationship of tender caring and faithful love would characterize the environment of a family. It was that but more. The interpenetration of persons in the Godhead provides a magnificent understanding of humankind's relationship to God, and who we are as created in His image. Sexuality is core to our personhood. It is far more than a conjugal act. God created us to enjoy an intimate, committed relationship to Him, which is demonstrated in the sexual relationship of a man and woman in a comr 'tted marital

---

15   John Stott, *Decisive Issues Facing Christians Today* (Old Tappan, New Jersey: Fleming H. Revell Company,1984 and 1990), 259.

relationship. God sought time and conversation with Adam and Eve. He walked with them every day in joyful, unhindered companionship. When sin entered the picture, the innocence and openness of the relationship was cut off and Adam and Eve attempted to hide themselves from God.

Behind the sin was the seductive act of Satan, the father of lies. The lie has perpetrated into two extremes. On one hand, sex is presented by a godless culture as a fabulous sensual experience, a sport that is genital focused. On the opposite extreme, the church has barricaded sex behind locked doors and approached with don't do it or you might get pregnant, STDs or AIDS. The former is demonstrably hollow; the latter is demonstrably shallow and absent an understanding of the true nature of sex as core to one's personhood.

In the unity of God each person shares the same essence, or substance, while maintaining personal distinction. In the beginning God said that *'a man will leave his father and mother and be united to his wife, and they will become one flesh'* (Genesis 1:24). Two Hebrew words are translated 'one' in our English Bibles. Here it is a word referring to a composite one ('echâd); the two are not only one in a sexual unity, but one in a spiritual and emotional unity. In the *Shema* (Deuteronomy 6:4), 'the question of diversity within unity has theological implications. Some scholars have felt that, though 'one' is singular, the usage of the word allows for the doctrine of the Trinity.'[16] The union of man and woman in marriage reflects the union of the Godhead. When Jesus took our sin and was made

16   R. Laird Harrris, ed., *Theological Wordbook of the Old Testament* (Chicago: Moody Press, 1980), Vol. 1, 30, item 61.

sin, the Father turned away from the Son causing Jesus to cry
in desperation, 'My God, my God, why have you forsaken me?'
At that moment the Triune God was fractured because of sin.
Paul declared that Jesus, who was sinless became sin that we
might be made righteous in Him (2 Corinthians 5:21). Sexual
sin destroys the unique intimacy sex was designed to portray. [17]

The other word for 'one' carries the concept of a tender,
unique relationship, an only begotten. God told Abraham
(Genesis 22:2) to take his 'only' (*yâchîyd*) son, meaning his
unique son of promise whom he loved for a sacrificial offering,
rather than the previous son of human determination, Ishmael.
Harris wrote of Isaac and as an 'only' son: "It is tempting to
see here the idea of 'incomparable' and 'without parallel'
anticipating the Messiah in His 'unique' relationship to the
Father who claims him as…'my beloved Son' (Mt. 3:17;
17:5)."[18] Marriage is to reflect the unique relationship of the
Trinity of distinctness of persons yet unity of purpose and
tender loving relationship. Just as God joyfully anticipated His
walk with Adam and Eve each evening, so husbands and wives
are to joyfully anticipate time together in intimacy of which sex
is a climactic expression.

When Israel and Judah chose to turn away from God
to worship the manufactured deities of Canaanite fertility
religions, the only descriptive that would fit the heinous sin
was adultery and prostitution. It was the betrayal of trust and

---

17   See Appendix A for listing of Scripture references to ᵃᵈᵘ᷄tery an᷄
prostitution.

18   Harris, 372, item 858.

integrity that occurs when either a wife or husband shacks up with someone else.

The three persons of the Trinity have one will and one emotion. All three persons love the same and hate the same, they will the same. There is no competition for supremacy or difference of choice. What the Father willed, the Son carried out, and what the Son provided in His saving work the Holy Spirit effects in the life of the believer. This interpenetration and unity is based on integrity, the foundation of trust. Without trust there cannot be the long-term relationship of intimacy between humanity and God, which was God's purpose in creating humans in the first place. (*In love he predestined us to be adopted as his sons through Jesus Christ* Ephesians 1:5). The Father determined to have a family of sons and daughters on whom He could lavish His love and from whom He would receive a love-commitment of loyalty, trust and constant communion. In addition, sexual intimacy is the most intense and spiritual experience available to mortals, which is why it is surrounded with mystery. Sex as an expression of integrity is a part of the nature of God; it was not an after-thought or an accident. God made humans sexual as a part of His image. Humankind is designed for relationship, the apex of which is the sexual union of a husband and wife.

Sex demands integrity to produce the end result that we long for. One of the most sexual characters of the Bible had a lot to say about integrity. Did he have any?

*S*ex, like God's relationship to His people, is about integrity, not only pleasure, or sport, or a power move to prove either femininity or masculinity. Sex is intensely social and intensely personal.

4

SEX IS ABOUT INTEGRITY

We are now at the end of our enquiry. It is just about two hundred years since the secular intellectuals began to replace the old clerisy as the guides and mentors of mankind (Paul Johnson).[19]

One of the most powerful Hebrew words of the Old Testament is *hesed* (חֶסֶד *chêsêd*). It was used of keeping legal obligations and communicates the integrity of God in keeping His promises and obligations. Some translations of the word include: 'unfailing love,' 'kindness,' 'goodness', 'loyal love,' 'stubborn faithfulness,' and 'loving-kindness.' In secular terminology it described 'a man's faithfulness to his treaty obligations', and in reference to God, to His 'faithfulness to the testament and its promises.'[20] *Hesed* served as the basis of the testament, God's promises to His people, for an agreement has value only if those entering it have the integrity to keep it. Balaam, though in the end he proved to be a false, money-hungry prophet hit the bulls eye when he declared (Numbers

---

19   Johnson, 342.
20   J. Barton Payne, *The Theology of the Older Testament* (Grand Rapids, Michigan: Zondervan Publishing House, 1962), 162.

24:19): "God is not a man that he should lie, nor a son of man, that he should change his mind. Does he speak and then not act? Does he promise and not fulfill?" Because of His integrity people can place their trust in God and His statements as given to us in the Bible.

Biblical and subsequent history proves that God has been faithful to His word, but humanity has utterly failed. God's relationship to His people is based upon an agreement He entered into with full integrity. He utilized covenants, or testaments, to establish His commitments. He promised to give Abraham a land for his descendants who would be as plentiful as the sand of the sea and the stars of heaven. It was a unilateral agreement that did not require any specific action from Abraham other than to leave his homeland and travel via camel and donkeys, leading stock and children, from the Fertile Crescent to Canaan. Some 400 years later, Israel, having been released from slavery in Egypt, took possession of the land the LORD had given centuries before. The conquest of Canaan proved the faithfulness of God. Faithfulness is the artesian fountain of God's unfailing love. "The Hebrew root that is involved is *aman*, 'Amen,' which means 'to be steady, or firm.' From this root are derived the two nouns *emuna*, 'faithfulness,' and *emeth*, 'truth.'"[21] Moses encountered these qualities when he was alone with God on Mt. Sinai. He longed for God to reveal Himself. And God responded: "The LORD [Yahweh, the personal God of the covenant], the LORD, the compassionate and gracious God, slow to anger, abounding in love *(hesed)* and faithfulness *(emeth)*" (Exodus 34:6).

---

21   Payne, *Ibid.*

Centuries later, David spoke repeatedly of the unfailing love and faithfulness of the LORD. "All the ways of the LORD are loving *(hesed)* and faithful *(emeth)* for those who keep the demands of his covenant" (Psalm 25:10). "For great is your [unfailing] love, reaching to the heavens; your faithfulness to the skies" (57:10). "But you O Lord, are a compassionate and gracious God, slow to anger and abounding in [unfailing] love and faithfulness" (86:15). Solomon told God: "You showed [unfailing] love to my father David because he was faithful [*emeth*] to you and righteous and upright in heart" (1 Kings 3:6). How could David be referred to as righteous when he had committed adultery and murder? It is a superlative witness to the faithfulness of a forgiving God who gives people a new start. God looked to His people to reflect back to Him the same qualities He gave to them which, as in David's case and so the rest of humanity, does not require moral perfection. Rather, it requires coming to a forgiving God who is faithful to His promises. Because of the character of God's trustworthiness, He is referred to as a 'rock,' a 'refuge,' and the 'horn of salvation.'

The LORD promised to be their God and they were to be His people, which included He would be the sole object of worship. When they willfully, brazenly, and arrogantly broke the agreement, it was an act of adultery and prostitution. Religion centers on the integrity of God in keeping His promises and His people keeping theirs to Him. As previously cited, God said to His people: "I gave you my solemn oath and entered into a covenant with you...and you became mine" (Ezekiel 16:8). He kept His part of the covenant, the people did not.

When God gave Moses the Ten Commandments, He prohibited His people from worshiping or bowing down to any other god because he was a jealous God (Exodus 20:5). Later in verse 14 His name is Jealous. That is the language of a lover wanting to protect His loved one from anything that would harm. His judgment was incisive and powerful to Israel and Judah, but came after centuries of their persistent violation of covenanted love despite repeated prophetic warnings of judgment to come.

Sex, like God's relationship to His people, is about integrity, not only pleasure, or sport, or a power move to prove either femininity or masculinity. Sex is intensely social and intensely personal. It can only express integrity when two people are free and choose to unite their personal integrity into one being. Otherwise, sex is simply a social/physical act of pleasure that leads to 'there must be something more than this.'

After David's affair with Bathsheba was exposed, he asked the Lord to 'have mercy upon me, O God, according to your unfailing love, *hesed*' (Psalm 51:1). Hebrew poetry restated the thought of the first couplet in the following couplet. It is so in this psalm. In the next lines of verse one David appealed to God's 'great compassion' (NIV), or 'tender mercies' (KJV). This second word, *racham*, comes from a root meaning to fondle and includes the tender care of a mother for her baby. David's hope of forgiveness was based on a God who is faithful to His covenant in the face of human failure, and to a God whose tender love is compared to the fondling of lovers as they explore their love, or to the watchful eye of a mother for the baby she carries.

Today's practice of a trial sexual relationship 'to see
if we're compatible' violates the very nature of God who
has covenanted with us to love us in our failures and self-
centeredness. David knew he could rely on the integrity of the
stubborn faithfulness of God to forgive his belligerent lust.
Hosea is a graphic personal illustration of loyal love. His love
for his adulterous wife and her lustful wanderings after lovers
baffles the most romantic mind. How could he take her back?
The same way God restored a people to Himself who had
played the prostitute with other gods. "I will betroth you to
me forever; I will betroth you in righteousness and justice, in
love [*hesed*] and compassion [*racham*]. I will betroth you in
faithfulness..." (Hosea 2:19). To buy into today's moral sludge
where commitment is non-existent and fidelity is only to our
own convenience is to be a part of Israel, not to be like Christ.

God's integrity is the foundation of His relationship to
those He created in His own image, and therefore, integrity
must be the foundation of all human relationships of which
marriage is the superlative. With integrity in place, God used
the sexual image to convey the intimacy of His love and
interaction with His people. His call to us is to enjoy intimacy
with Him. As referred to previously, the same word chosen
to speak of sexual relations, 'Adam **knew** his wife Eve and
she conceived,' is used to speak of God's relation to people.
After Moses' death, it was recorded: "Since then, no prophet
has risen in Israel like Moses, whom the LORD **knew** face to
face..." (Deuteronomy 34:10). The same word is also used of
family and other social personal relationships. Likewise we are
to 'know' God. When God first came to the young boy Samuel,

the account reads, "Samuel did not yet **know** the LORD" (1 Samuel. 3:7). After having written dramatically of the depth of God's omniscience, David expressed his longing for God to know him fully: "Search me, O God, and **know** my heart; test me and **know** my anxious thoughts" (Psalm. 139:23).

The tabernacle where God desired to meet with His people carries the same imagery. The word for 'meet' (*ya'adh*) means appoint, fix, betroth, given in marriage, or come together. God longs for an intimate meeting with His 'beloved'.

The New Testament synonym for *hesed* is *charis* (grace) and provides a deeper insight into God bringing people into an intimate relationship with Him. God lovingly calls people in His new covenant to enjoy intimacy with Him as a free gift. We do not earn the right to know Him. We do not initiate coming to Him. He initiates with us as the groom to the bride. The grace of God is stated to us as a promise. In the same way, God's promise of prosperity and a land was given to Abraham, Isaac, and Jacob, so His promise of forgiveness and eternal life is given in and through Jesus Christ. Through integrity God kept His promises and the Israelites entered Canaan. There is still a land and a people today some 3,500 years later. God's integrity also has provided the ultimate people of God, Jew and Gentile, and the ultimate possession of a land, heaven, in the new testament of the blood of Jesus of Nazareth. In Him there is both forgiveness and eternal life as gifts of grace.

The Abrahamic promise issued in a testament in which God's people were to obey His law and worship only the LORD, and that only in the prescribed ritual. Their failure to keep the covenant through spiritual adultery resulted in God's avowing them 'not loved,' and 'not my people' as Hosea declared.

The grace promise provided the benefits of forgiveness and eternal life in becoming children of God without human obligation. Repentance of sin and faith in the Lord Jesus Christ are the only requisites to receive the promise. Further, the grace promise provided spiritual regeneration and change of heart to empower faithful and holy living that was not a part of the Old Testament.

A complementary word to *charis* is *agapē* (love). It does not refer primarily to emotion, but to willful behavior arising not out of obligation but out of the 'royal' law now written in our hearts. One described *agapē* as 'not a hunger that needs to be filled, but a fullness that gives away.' A person's love is demonstrated in how they treat another. God loves us and is eager to penetrate our lives with His saving grace as we respond to His tender invitation to come to Him. In calling us, He accepts us with our failings, sins, and weaknesses. But He is not content for us to continue in former behaviors. He will only have a bride that is pure. He cleanses our sins and puts His Spirit in us to give us life and power to live pleasing to Him. It is all God's saving action given in grace. Our level of acceptance before God is elevated to equal the acceptance that Jesus Himself enjoys with the Father.

An obvious reason for the use of the sexual metaphor is that everyone can understand what God is saying. People have never had a problem catching on to sex. As the Broadway musical stated, it's doing what comes naturally. Naturally, because that is how God created us. Yet, the not-so-obvious fact is that for sex to meet its highest expectations and not produce destruction, it must be expressed within the context of integrity, loyal love and faithfulness to a covenant. Marriage, as established by God and recorded in Genesis, predated the Law. As cultures developed and civilizations were created, covenantal marriage became an economic contract. Economic power became a determinate factor in marriage, and marriage degenerated into special cases of slavery contracts between a man, a woman, and God.

The marriage that analogizes the union of Christ and the church as His bride is the marriage of faith, pre-law and post-law. Salvation is not the result of the promises to Jacob the deceiver and the father of law, but of Abraham the faithful, the father of faith. Since freedom to have personal integrity comes only through Christ, it is not possible for two to be married in faith outside of Christ. Paul stated that if an unbelieving partner chose to remain, he/she would be conformed to the integrity of the believer (1 Corinthians 7:14). Integrity can be achieved in spiritually divided marriages if these factors exist. Two partners are to promise each other to love, cherish and care for one another. Those verbal statements are to be backed by integrity.

From a biblical perspective, sex is more than an orgasm, it is a union of souls that are spiritual beings first, and physical beings second. Without faith, sex is only a social/physical interaction of two humans. While the superiority of the spirit is true in all of human experience, it is nowhere more dominant than in the sexual. Because humans are born spiritually dead, separated from God, we easily miss what should be obvious. The believer who has been made alive by the Spirit's personal indwelling presence still has an inside pull to the old life. So believers, too, have a natural bent to view sex only as a physically pleasurable act. He or she lives in an orgasmic culture where sex is viewed only through a sensual lens. To simply say 'no' or to protect from unwanted pregnancies and STDs has not curbed exploitation at ever younger ages. Is it time for going a little deeper in our thinking of why God made us sexual?

How does God fit into the picture of human sex? Is there sex in the Trinity?

No lies are more prevalent than the mating language used to get another into bed. That is not love. Yet human love can have the same integrity of God's love because of His saving power to change us. We can do better than live on the superficial level of sexual lust.

5

SEX AND THE
CHARACTER OF GOD

God is Holy

*Everything is connected, and everything points beyond itself—
especially sex (Peter Kreeft)*[22]

*One of the ends for which sex was created was to symbolize to
us the hidden things of God. One of the functions of human
marriage is to express the nature of the union between Christ
and the church.* (C. S. Lewis) [23]

*The neo-orthodox theologian Barth viewed the gift of sexuality
as fundamental to the image of God which humans reflect.
Barth, and many since, have suggested that human sexuality
reflects the differentiation of persons within the Godhead and
God's intimately relational nature…. Thus our sexual natures
reflect the nature of the Creator of the universe.*[24]

Holy is that quality of God that distinguishes Him from
everything else, whether religious deity, humankind, or matter.

---

22   Kreeft: *ibid.*, page 2.
23   C. S. Lewis, quoted by Kreeft, *ibid.*
24   S. L. Jones, "Sexuality," David G. Benner, Peter C. Hill, *Baker
Encyclopedia of Psychology* (Grand Rapids, Mich.: Baker Books 1985), 1065.

It is the characteristic that enables Him to perfectly love what is pure and hate what is impure. The pure is always good, impure is always bad. Purity always benefits people, impurity always damages. God has never been confused about either one. He doesn't debate with anyone; He is, instead, the One who makes up the rules that define good and evil, right and wrong. The Bible lists specific attitudes and behaviors that are pure and others that are impure. Impure behaviors are said to be sinful behavior that misses the target of purity and goodness. Sin, therefore always has negative results in human experience. The Bible expresses this negative as death. God is without sin in thought, motive, or act. As a holy God His lists of good and evil are not arbitrary. They define what is pure and impure, and what will hurt or help His creation. It is only in the realm of humanity that there is any challenge to God's rules about life. The animal world is controlled by basic instincts placed within by nature's God. Animals do not consciously decide to accept or reject those instincts. Since human beings are in the image of God, they alone have the ability to consciously accept or reject submission to the rules of behavior God has established.

The Law God gave the Hebrews has a list of specific regulations related to sex. Heading the list is the seventh of the Ten Commandments to not commit adultery. Deuteronomy 22:22 establishes death by stoning for both man and woman in adultery. In verses 25-29 if a man rapes a girl pledged to be married to another in a remote place he is to be stoned, but not her. However, if she is not engaged to someone, he must pay the girl's father a financial payment and marry her. Following in verse 30, a man cannot marry his father's wife. Exodus

22:1 discusses a man seducing a virgin and verse 19 calls for death when someone has sex with an animal. Deuteronomy 23:9-11 states cleanliness rules when a man has a nocturnal emission. Verse 17 forbids a man or woman to become a temple prostitute. Further expressions of sexual sin are listed in the statement of curses in Deuteronomy 27:20-23. With these various sins listed, nothing is said in either Testament about masturbation, which seems to indicate that God does not view that behavior as a sin. The only possible reference was when Onan, the son of Judah, ejaculated his seed on the ground rather than impregnate his brother's wife and so raise up an heir to Er, his brother (Genesis 38:6-10). "What he did was wicked in the LORD's sight; so he put him to death also." There are other reasons habitual masturbation should not be indulged in, but sin is evidently not one of them. This list of restrictions on sexual behavior clarifies what God views as unholy and therefore not to be part of the behavior of His people.

God established boundaries for sexual expression for our good. His lines of circumference were not arbitrarily established but were based upon His perfect knowledge of what is good and beneficial, and what is evil and destructive. However, the sin-driven nature of humans demands to break the boundaries. A television commercial illustrated this. The art class teacher encouraged the children to color within the lines, for the 'lines are our friends.' The boundary-friend message was repeated several times until finally one student, in frustration, scribbled all over the paper. The ad promoted a sport utility vehicle that could handle off-road terrain, but the message of breaking the boundaries because those lines bring frustration was clear enough. Morally, breaking the boundaries doesn't bring fulfillment in the long term. There may be momentary ecstasy or thrill, but sin always wounds the individual and society. The paycheck of sin is death, but the gift of God is life (Romans 6:23).

Why the boundary of a heterosexual, life-long marriage for sexual intimacy? Because that type of relationship is best for us and for society as a whole. What if a person chooses to reject those lines and scribble all over the sexual page? The holiness of God requires sin, the breaking of the boundaries, to be paid for. We pay for it lots of ways, but God Himself ended up taking the full brunt of the penalty instead of us so He could rescue people from their own deliberate choices of destruction. That is grace.

A holy God has called His people to share in His distinctiveness, so He invites them to be holy as He is holy (Leviticus 11:44; 1 Peter 1:15-16). In Deuteronomy, God required His people to distinguish themselves from the rest of the people of the world by certain behaviors. The basis was their being set apart to belong to the LORD. "You are a people holy to the LORD your God. Out of all the peoples on the face of the earth, the LORD has chosen you to be his treasured possession" (Deuteronomy 14:2-3). Moses' sermons in Deuteronomy proscribe the lines within which the holy people were to live so that they could enjoy blessing, prosperity, and triumph over their enemies. God's people are responsible to demonstrate unfailing love and faithfulness, too. Lasting happiness comes from staying within God's lines because they are there for a reason—our good!

Compare it to buying a new car, a privilege I've enjoyed a couple of times. Every new car comes with an Owner's Manual that tells the owner how to take care of their vehicle. Most manufacturers recommend oil and filter changes every 5-10,000 miles, depending on the kind of driving a person does and the type of oil used. I have talked with service managers who have told me of owners who totally disregarded the instructions going 25-30,000 miles without an oil change. What happened in those cases? The warranty was nullified and sometimes the engine received severe damage. Is the Owner's Manual for a car a wet blanket book? Hardly. It is written to inform the owner how the auto was made and how it should be taken care of in order to get the best performance from it. So it is with the sexual boundaries established by God. He made us, and He has given an Owner's Manual to enable us to get the most out of life. There may be a certain 'gusto' gained by hooking up because of the excitement of flirting and exploration. For many males sex is conquest. Females may be looking for validation of attractiveness. Whatever the reason for a weekend tryst, it doesn't produce the long-term happiness or intimacy a person is searching for. Delayed gratification is foreign to today's vocabulary, but it can be the path to greater happiness and wholeness.[25]

---

25   Tim Chaddick, pastor of Reality LA, "Ministering to Millennials about Sex," addresses the why question in an excellent video interview: https://www.barna.org/barna-update/millennials/684-q-a-with-tim-chaddick-ministering-to-millennials-about-sex#.VEbD6hY0upg.

In addition, there is a dignity in belonging to God that is
reflected in the way a child of God behaves. We might compare
it to belonging to the House of Windsor in England, the royal
family. In 1992, the royal family was rocked by sexual scandals
and the revelation of both princes' cold treatment of their
wives. In a television drama of Andrew's saga with Fergie,
he said to her, "We have to give something back, Fergie." He
meant the privilege of being in the royal family carried an
obligation to the people of Britain. If that applies to a human
royal family, how much more appropriate it is for God to
expect His family to behave in a way that demonstrates their
attachment to Him.

God's distinctive character is one thing, but He is also
defined as love. How does that fit the subject?

God is Love

Love is not something God has. It is something that He
is (1 John 4:8). That love is more than emotion, though it
embraces and elevates emotion. God's love is pictured in words
like 'faithful' and 'longsuffering'. The expression of God's
faithfulness was not limited to the abstract of philosophical
thinking. God promised Abraham that He would give him and
His innumerable descendants a land with defined boundaries.
Centuries went by before the Israelites, rescued from Egyptian
slavery, were released through the Exodus and entered into
that Promised Land. It was God's unfailing love that caused
Him to keep His covenant with Abraham. The character quality
empowering that unfailing love was the faithfulness of God.
The very name God used to speak of Himself, the LORD (all

upper case to represent YHWH) carries a basic meaning of one who exists and is faithful.[26] Moses knew God's character when on Mt. Sinai God said to him: "The LORD, the LORD, the compassionate and gracious God, slow to anger, abounding in unfailing love and faithfulness" (Exodus 34:6). He proved His faithfulness in concrete experience when He empowered the Israelites to enter and conquer Canaan. He could be trusted. True love is trustworthy. Moses recorded God's clear demand for the sole worship and loyalty of His people. "You must worship no other gods, for the LORD, whose name is jealous, is a God who is jealous about his relationship with you" (Exodus 34:14-17, NLT).

Can you imagine what it would be like to attempt worshipping a god who was **un**faithful? If you trusted him to do what he promised one minute, could you trust him to be there for you the next? Such a being would not be worthy of trust. Unfortunately, many people have had spouses or lovers like that. Some feel trapped by their own sense of faithfulness to stay with an unfaithful partner, even as Hosea did. Spouses who are both faithful to each other have a security that enables them to look at their differences, learn from each other, grow

---

26   *The LORD.* The Hebrew for this name is *Yahweh* (often incorrectly spelled 'Jehovah'; see note on Dt 28:58). It means 'He is' or 'He will be' and is the third-person form of the verb translated 'I will be' in v. 12 and 'I AM' in v. 14. When God speaks of himself he says, 'I AM,' and when we speak of him we say, 'He is.' [NIV study notes on Exod. 3:15]. "Scripture speaks of the Tetragrammaton as 'this glorious and fearful name' (Deut 28:58) or simply 'the name (Lev 24:11). But it connotes God's nearness, his concern for man and the revelation of his redemptive covenant." [R. Laird Harris, Gleason L. Archer, Jr., Bruce K. Waltke, *Theological Wordbook of the Old Testament* (Chicago: Moody Press, 1980) Vol. 1, 212.]. "It expresses the eternity and immutability of the divine nature, and the faithfulness of God to all his purposes and promises." [William Wilson, *Old Testament Word Studies*, (Grand Rapids, Michigan: Kregel Publications, 1978), 259].

and mature. Such trust goes on into old age. Nothing is more beautiful. At the same time, nothing is more tragic than people whose word means nothing and whose sexual exploits have given them a lot of thrills but no lasting happiness, no life-long companionship in which they grow old together. In the coming years a twenty-fifth, let alone a fiftieth, wedding anniversary will be a unique event.

One of the primary Hebrew words translated 'faithful' carries with it the idea of security. God's faithfulness to His promises gives security to His people whether it applies to the great issue of eternity or to daily needs for sustenance. It is found twenty-two times in the Psalms and is often associated with unfailing love (*hesed*). The psalmist assures us: "For the word of the Lord is right and true; he is faithful in all he does" (Psalm 33:4). God's word on sexual boundaries is right and true. Security is found in staying within the lines. "I will sing of the Lord's great love *(hesed)* forever; with my mouth I will make your faithfulness known through all generations. I will declare that your love (*hesed*) stands firm forever, that you established your faithfulness (*'emuwnah*) in heaven itself" (Psalm 89:1-2). God's love is commitment to His promises: blessing for obedience, justice for scribbling all over His page and discarding the Owner's Manual. His love is as secure as heaven itself. Therefore, God's people have assurance that in obeying His word, they can't go wrong. Trust does not exist in a vacuum, it requires the object be worthy of trust, whether divine or human. The greatest offense to a person is a false god eliciting trust and then not performing in the ultimate sense of eternity. Satan is the deceiver whose goal is destruction. False religion, religion that promises some form of eternal life but doesn't actually deliver, is spiritual rape.

Trust is the foundation of all relationships: whether two people, a community of people in a locale, or state and national government. All over the world, citizens no longer trust their governments. Cynicism and distrust have spawned anger, violence, and revolution as people have lashed out against the repeated failures of their leaders to do what is right. Charles Colson commented:

> We forget sometimes what a fragile thing the American experiment in government is. It works only when the governed and the governors share a common goal, a common moral standard. Philosophers have always argued that a political order rests upon a moral order, a shared set of beliefs and values. What binds society together is the trust that we will all regulate our conduct according to an agreed-upon moral framework. The problem is that since the 1960's the notion of a common moral framework has steadily eroded. A radical individualism, rooted in existentialism, has taken hold in our culture, leaving many people reluctant to say that there are any universal norms for conduct....

> A second consequence of radical individualism is a loss of trust. In any relationship, trust is based not merely on people's good will—we all know that can fluctuate. Instead, trust results from knowing the other person is committed to a shared standard binding on us both.[27]

Erotic love by its nature knows no integrity, only grasping for satisfaction. That is the love of MTV, the soaps, and many

---

27   *USA Today*, Sept. 24, 1992, "Opinion USA."

movies. Eros can't be trusted. Love, that is *agapē*, and trust are synonymous.

Covenants and vows in the marriage ceremony reflect the integrity of God in His promises. A man and woman stand before a minister who represents God, and promise to be true to each other in all of the good and bad events of life. Many ceremonies will have two parts: a statement of covenant, and vows. A sample covenant reads: "Before God and these witnesses, will you [groom's full name] take [bride's full name] to be your bride? Will you love and comfort her, honor and keep her and, in joy and sorrow, preserve with her this bond, holy and unbroken, until the coming of our Lord Jesus Christ, or as long as you both shall live?" The groom is to respond with 'I will.' The theology of the ceremony broadens the public statements of commitment to include the witnesses of the wedding party, the congregation attending, and the minister as a representative of God before whom the covenantal oath is given. The exchange of vows follows the covenantal pledge with integrity as the bottom line of the ceremony. These commitments are symbolized by the circles of rings. Can each be trusted to keep their word, or will certain contingencies arise giving a loophole to jump out? Obviously, with no fault divorce laws, one's word before a minister or justice of the peace doesn't mean much. Malachi stated the sacredness of these vows. The prophet rebuked the people's tearful pleading with God to bring blessing to them because they were bringing Him offerings. But God paid no attention to them. How often do we think that if we go to church and drop a ten dollar bill, God is going to leap with joy? Why did He reject them?

"You ask, 'Why?' It is because the LORD is acting as the witness between you and the wife of your youth, because you have broken faith with her, though she is your partner, the wife of your marriage covenant. Has not the LORD made them one? In flesh and spirit they are his. And why one? Because he was seeking godly offspring. So guard yourself in your spirit, and do not break faith with the wife of your marriage covenant" (Malachi 2:14-15).

Malachi went further to explain that when God created male and female and established marriage, He made the two people one. Sex unites both flesh and spirit. Why, asked Malachi. The answer is that God sought a family that reflected His own nature. Malachi's conclusion: "So guard yourself in your spirit, and do not break faith with the wife of your youth."

One exhaustive study by two sociologists, James Paterson and Peter Kim, found Americans are habitual liars.[28] Sexual license makes people liars. The young man whose hot breath whispers 'I love you' means little more than I want you to meet my immediate sexual needs. No lies are more prevalent than the mating language used to get another into bed. That is not love. Yet human love can have the same integrity of God's love because of His saving power to change us. We can do better than live on the superficial level of sexual lust. We are of far greater value than an animal for we are made in the image of God. Lack of integrity makes our vows and covenants meaningless. We really are saying 'to have and to hold from this day forward' until I change my mind. That blatantly limits acceptance of another person, puts trust in the closet, reduces

---

28   James Paterson and Peter Kim, *The Day America Told the Truth* (New York: Prentice Hall Press, 1991).

relationship to a matter of performance to please another, and denies any reality of God's personal presence in our lives. If one accepts the 'exception clause' of Matthew 19:9 of adultery being cause for divorce, it is because sexual immorality is a violation of trust, the foundation of the relationship, and the integrity, and faithfulness that it produces.

Sexual immorality breaks down the inner character of a person more quickly than any other type of activity. Sex is part of the core of a person's heart. To be dishonest there leads to dishonesty in many other areas. God made us as sexual beings and gave sex its enormous power to allow a husband and wife to enjoy lifelong pleasure and intimacy. No sin brings greater spiritual consequences than sexual sin. It sears our consciences, causing a moral perversion in which wrong is justified and even made to be spiritual, 'I've prayed about it and the Lord assured me it is okay.' There may have been an inner voice of assurance, but it was not God's voice. He doesn't contradict His Word. In a message to the thousands of teens at a Youth for Christ convention at Winona Lake in 1956 that I personally attended as a college student, Billy Graham stated that no sin sears the conscience faster than sexual sin.

Proverbs warns the young man (chapter 5) to not be enticed to the prostitute's bed. Solomon, who understood sex quite well, warned of the long-term consequences of immorality. A man gives away his strength to one who is cruel (9), wastes his wealth (10), and "at the end of your life you will groan, when your flesh and body are spent. You will say, 'How I hated discipline! How my heart spurned correction! I would not obey my teachers or listen to my instructors'" (11-13). His advice was to 'drink water from your own cistern [meaning wife].... May your fountain be blessed, and may you rejoice in the wife of your youth. A loving doe, a graceful deer—may her breasts satisfy you always, may you ever be captivated by her love" (15-19). Contrast that with American life where one in five Americans lose their virginity before the age of 13, and "religion plays no role in shaping more than half of all Americans' opinions on such issues as sexuality and birth control."[29] The American public has chosen to ignore the wisdom given 3,000 years ago. God's love is faithful love. Love can be trusted. Trust is evidenced in the very nature of the Godhead.

God is Triune

The persons of the triune God relate to one another without deception or rivalry. There is total openness and trust in the Godhead. Contrast that harmonious picture with the intrigue, contention, and competition among the Grecian gods and goddesses. God designed a husband and wife to experience the safety and freedom of relationship that reflects of His own personal existence. Jesus' high priestly prayer in John 17 expressed the desire that believers would have the same oneness with each other as was enjoyed within the Godhead. If that was to be the case on the social level, it is critically more important in marriage with sexual intimacy expressing unity in its highest form.

Sex, as a reflection of the nature of God, takes us into another level of consideration. Sex is central to who and what we are, not a side-spur. God used sex as a metaphor to

29   *U.S. News and World Report,* 10 June 1991, 64.

demonstrate that it is core to who we are as His creation. When they turned from Him, He accused them of adultery. Why? Part of the answer lies in the nature of God. God is a relational being as a triune God. There isn't a male and female and child in the Godhead. Yet there is perfect intimacy in open giving and sharing among the persons.

"*Perichorēsis* is a term relating to the doctrine of the Trinity, often also referred to by the Latin term *circumincessio*. The basic notion is that all three persons of the Trinity mutually share in the life of the others, so that none is isolated or detached from the actions of the others."[30] Another writer used the word 'interpenetration' to define *perichorēsis*. While there is no thought or reference to sexual activity in this term, it does communicate the level of intimacy enjoyed by the persons of the Trinity, a true interpenetration, a dance of intimacy. "The concept of *perichorēsis* allows the individuality of the persons to be maintained, while insisting that each person shares in the life of the other two. An image often used to express this idea is that of 'a community of being.'"[31] As this description is linked to *homoousios* (of the same substance) the image is deepened. The Nicene Creed declares that Jesus is 'of one substance with the Father'. Although the Bible is clear in stating the Father is God, the Son is God and the Holy Spirit is God, it also states that God is one (Deuteronomy 6:4). Each person of the Trinity is a distinct person. Augustine took the above three statements a step further and emphasized that the Father is NOT the Son,

---

30   Alister E. McGrath, *Christian Theology: An Introduction* (University of Oxford: Blackwell Publishing, 2007), 492.
31   *Ibid.*, 251.

the Son is NOT the Spirit and the Spirit is NOT the Father, yet there is one God.

Homoousios describes the reality that the three persons have one mind, one will (one in action), and are one emotionally (all perfectly love the right and hate sin and evil). Our previous reference to Genesis 2:24 stated that a man and woman became one flesh through sexual union. That oneness reaches its highest expression as a couple works to develop unity of mind, will and begin to respond emotionally in the same way. This is why Paul emphasized to the carnal believers in Corinth that they were not to have sex with a prostitute. "Do you not know that he who unites himself with a prostitute is one with her in body? For it is said, 'The two will become one flesh.' But he who unites himself with the Lord is one with him in spirit. Flee from sexual immorality" (1 Corinthians 6:16-18a).

God created a capacity for procreation that incorporated the core of His own existence as a relational God. He made sex more than a mere procreative act as it is in the animal kingdom. Sex is a means of expressing His nature as a relational God by designing a man and woman to become one flesh, welded together in intimacy of spirit expressed in the conjugal act. The reason recreational sex falls short is because it doesn't meet the longing for intimacy that sex is designed to express. It degenerates to the level of sensual pleasure only.

Intimacy is a relational issue. Relationships, in the home and society, must be based upon the integrity of the persons involved who keep their promises. The Trinity conveys that God is a relational being. Each person is faithful to the other and needs nothing outside their mysterious relationship for fulfillment. God is the only being who is self-sufficient. Because the intimacy of the Godhead is complete and perfect, He needs no one else to fill a void. The God of the Bible does not consort with other gods in order to fulfill a longing. He is fullness and gives to us out of His fullness needing nothing from us. When a marriage enjoys social and spiritual intimacy, there is no need to search for completeness by pursuing sex with other partners. Theologian, Karl Barth, "viewed sexuality as fundamental to the image of God which humans reflect. Barth and many since have suggested that human sexuality reflects the differentiation of persons within the Godhead and God's intimately relational nature…. Thus our sexual natures reflect the nature of the Creator of the universe."[32] Part of that image is the ability to create, not in the absolute sense of God creating the universe out of nothing, but in the more limited sense of works of art, invention, imaginative thinking, and procreation itself. Through the sexual act and conception, another eternal soul is created. That must be the closest thing human beings can come to being like God. In the sexual act, the two separate physical people become "one flesh" (Genesis 2:24). That is an irreducible intimacy, and in the same way, a person who trusts Christ is joined to the Lord and becomes one spirit with Him (1 Corinthians 6:17).

Stanton Jones suggested the creative and integrative role of sex as an expression of the triune God: "We might also argue that sexuality was divinely created to experientially teach us important truths about the Godhead and our relationship

---

32   Jones, *Ibid.*

thereunto. As argued earlier, gender differential reflects God's differentiated personhood, and sexual union in marriage reflects the complementary truth of union across differentiation within the Godhead and between God and humankind."[33] Marriage enables us to understand the "male" and "female" aspects of God better. The metaphor of sex enables us to better understand God, His unity, love, and integrity.

Since God is a spirit, and humankind was made in His image, then they, too, are spiritual beings first, and physical beings, second. A. W. Tozer wrote:

> The I AM which is God is underived and self-existent; the "I Am" which is man is derived from God and dependent every moment upon His creative fiat for its continued existence. One is the Creator, high over all, ancient of days, dwelling in light unapproachable. The other is a creature and, though privileged beyond all others, is still but a creature, a pensioner on God's bounty and a suppliant before His throne.
>
> The deep-in human entity of which we speak is called in the Scriptures *the spirit of man*. "For what man knoweth the things of man, save the spirit of man which is in him? even so the things of God knoweth no man, but the Spirit of God" (1 Corinthians 2:11). As God's self-knowledge lies in the eternal Spirit, so man's self-knowledge is by his own spirit, and his knowledge of God is by the direct impression of the Spirit of God upon the spirit of man.
>
> The importance of all this cannot be overestimated as we think and study and pray. It reveals the essential spirituality of mankind. It denies that man is a creature having a spirit and declares that he is a spirit having a body. That which makes him a human being is not his

33   *Ibid.,* 1066.

body but his spirit, in which the image of God originally lay.[34]

The spiritual dimension distinguishes human sex from animal sex. To begin with random chance evolution from lower animal forms of life, does not give any basis to call people to sexual standards different from animals, and perhaps that is why some feel free to call sex a sport. The spirit is humanity's link with God, his creator and Savior. The spirit is the source of meaning and purpose. It directs values and priorities and behavior. Love is first spiritual, the meaningful commitment of two people to one another in a permanent relationship. It is the ultimate expression of acceptance and trust. Sex is to flow out of that spiritual fountain. Promiscuity is often an outgrowth of a spiritual vacuum, whether expressed in self-doubt, the groping for acceptance, or the desire to be attractive sexually and personally to others. Sex alone can never provide the personal commitment and security of acceptance. That is gained in the context of a loving life-long commitment in marriage. Sex is the seal of a spiritual commitment of two people. In the same way, loyalty to God in our sex lives is a basic symbol of commitment to God. When people behave like animals, they deny their spiritual roots and evidence they are dead on the inside. God's anger is unleashed upon sexual promiscuity because it is a violation of trust and an abuse of the most vulnerable area of human existence. We will look further at this in chapter eleven.

---

34   A. W. Tozer, *Man the Dwelling Place of God* (Camp Hill, PA: Christian Publications, 1966), 9.

The very beginning of a person's relationship with God is described through the use of sexual terminology. How does the Bible express the concept of regeneration or born again?

_____

Sexual immorality breaks down the inner character of a person more quickly than any other type of activity.

A s the Holy Spirit overshadowed Mary empowering her pregnancy, so the Holy Spirit brings to a person the life of God as the seed of the Word is implanted in the heart of the believer and she or he is born again.

6

SEXUAL REFERENCES IN SALVATION

Understanding the Christian Life through the Sexual Metaphor

The word 'regeneration' (paliggenesia) literally means 'a birth again,' a new birth. It refers to a renovation, a renewal, a restoration, a re-creation.[35]

We may define regeneration as the communication of divine life to the soul (John 3:5; 10:10, 28; 1 John 5:11-12), as the impartation of a new nature (2 Pet. 1:4) or heart (Jer. 24:7; Ezek. 11:19; 36:26), and the production of a new creation (2 Cor. 5:17; Eph. 2:10; 4:24).[36]

It is probing that the language used to describe God's work in bringing a person to Himself utilizes sexual reference in the words chosen. For example, in Jesus' encounter in John 3 with the religious leader, Nicodemus, He employed the metaphor of birth. Unless a person is born again, or from above, he cannot

---

35   Harold M. Freligh, *The Eight Pillars of Salvation* (Minneapolis, Minnesota: Bethany Fellowship, Inc., 1962), 56.
36   Henry Clarence Thiessen, *Introductory Lectures in Systematic Theology* (Grand Rapids, Michigan: Wm. B. Eerdmans Publishing Co, 1975), 367.

see the kingdom of God. Reproduction of species is a result
of male/female sexual activity. Why did Jesus choose that
metaphor? Again, word pictures are powerful communicators.
Everyone is a result of birth and most everyone has seen some
type of birth directly or indirectly.

In Matthew, Mark and Luke, the parable of the sower
is presented and explained. In that parable, the word for
"seed" is *sperma*, which appears forty-four times in the New
Testament. Strong defines that word as "something sown, that
is, seed (including male sperm). B. A. Demarest wrote in *The
Dictionary of New Testament Theology*: "In the parable of
the sower (Matt. 13:1-9, par. Mk. 4:1-9; Lk. 8:4-8) emphasis
rests upon the act of seed sowing which, on the basis of
Jesus' identification of the *sperma* with the 'Word of God', is
symbolic of the proclamation of the arrival of the kingdom."[37]
As the Holy Spirit overshadowed Mary empowering her
pregnancy, so the Holy Spirit brings to a person the life of God
as the seed of the Word is implanted in the heart of the believer
and she or he is born again.

In a direct correlation of imagery, John writes (1John 3:9):
"No one who is born of God will continue to sin, because
God's seed remains in him; he cannot go on sinning, because
he has been born of God." Demarest comments: "The Philonic
concept of the 'divine seed' is given a Christian interpretation
in 1 Jn. 3:9, where sperma signifies the divine principle of
life (the Spirit?) in the believer, which renders continuance in

---

37   Colin Brown, General Editor, *The New International Dictionary of New
Testament Theology* (Grand Rapids, Michigan: Zondervan Publishing House, 1978),
Vol. III, 522

sin incongruous. As the physical sperma was the generator of life in the physical order (Gen. 1:11 ff.), so the divine sperma becomes the fount and origin of life in the new order of recreated humanity."[38]

In the previously quoted article by Peter Kreeft, he wrote of the "circumincession of divine Persons in the Trinity." The word, "circumincession" refers in theology to the "existence of persons in one another." He wrote: "God is masculine to everything, from angels to prime matter."[39] A fundamental axiom of soteriology (the doctrine of salvation): God is the initiator and the human being responds. As light penetrates darkness, a holy God penetrates the darkened spirit of humankind to bring light and life. John wrote in the opening of his gospel: "in him was life, and that life was the light of men. The light shines in the darkness, but the darkness has not understood it" (John 1:4-5). Light penetrates darkness.

Kreeft commented: "As a man comes into a woman's body from without to impregnate her, God creates the universe from without and performs miracles in it from without. He is not The Force but The Face; not Earth spirit rising but Heavenly Father descending; not the ideal construct of man's mind but the Hound of Heaven. To speak of 'religion' as 'man's search for God,' if we speak of this God, is like speaking of the mouse's search for the cat (to steal an image from C. S. Lewis)."[40]

In the first biblical reference to marital intercourse, Genesis 4:1 states "Now Adam knew Eve his wife, and she conceived"

---

38   Brown, *Ibid.*, 524.
39   Kreeft, *ibid.*, 3.
40   *Ibid*, 3-4.

(ESV). "Knew" is used in a variety of ways in the Old Testament. When applied to human sex it describes marital sex, sodomy (Genesis 19:5) and rape (Judges 19:25). The text states that Adam knew Eve, not that Eve knew Adam. Adam initiated, Eve responded. A son was conceived and born. God initiates in the pursuit of lost humanity. His Spirit penetrates the human spirit and we are born again and receive spiritual life.

In his article, Kreeft is arguing for the priority of male priest, which is not the direction or purpose of this book. However, he states that "something as deliberate and distinctive and as all-pervasive in Scripture as God's he-ness is no mere accident." At stake is revelation, the very purpose of "which is to reveal something that we could not have come up with from our own opinions or ideologies, to correct them."

This speaks to the central idea of the sexual metaphor that it opens a window into the person of God that would otherwise be closed to us. Thus the role of the sexual metaphor is the revelation of God disclosing who He is.

In this vein, the church (all who are in Christ by faith) is called the Bride of Christ. The result of the marriage is the spiritual fruit of divine or eternal life, and the product of the marriage is holiness. In contrast, spiritual adultery is eternal death and the product is sinful behavior. It denies God's initiative and replaces it with human initiative in forming and pursuing gods of their own making. Again, Kreeft states it concisely: "The new birth—our salvation—comes from above, from without, from transcendence. We do not spiritually impregnate ourselves with salvation or divine life any more than we physically impregnate ourselves. Modernism, humanism, and naturalism amount to spiritual auto-eroticism, spiritual masturbation."[41]

The previous discussion brings us to one of the most important dynamics of the Christian life. At conversion when a person repents of sin and independence and places trust in the Lord Jesus Christ as Savior and Leader, two things take place. One, Jesus comes to inhabit the person's life by the Holy Spirit. As Paul clearly states we become the temples of the Spirit. "Don't you know that you yourselves are God's temple and that God's Spirit lives in you? (1 Corinthians 3:16). On that basis, he reasons we are not to be sexually promiscuous. "The body is not meant for sexual immorality, but for the Lord, and the Lord for the body.... Do you not know that your bodies are members of Christ himself? Shall I take the members of Christ and unite them with a prostitute? Never! Do you not know that he who unites himself with a prostitute is one with her in body? For it is said, 'The two will become one flesh.' But he who unites himself with the Lord is one with him in spirit" (1 Corinthians 6:13-17).

The second thing that occurs at conversion is the believer is placed in Christ. That is the believer's position that grants her or him the actual sinlessness and perfection of Jesus before a holy God. As incredible as it sounds, a child of God in Christ is seen by the Father as perfect and sinless as Jesus is. This is known as positional sanctification. Although that is awesomely true, we are not sinless now. The Holy Spirit lives in us to empower and prompt even push us to obey God. That means

41   *Ibid.*, 5.

placing our sinful nature (*sarx*, flesh) on the cross. The word "flesh" refers to the drive inside us that is against what God wants, and demands immediate gratification of physical drives and desires. The flesh or sinful nature is to be crucified as discussed later.

The conjugal relationship of a husband and wife is a metaphor of Christ in the believer and the believer in Christ. The frequent biblical expression is "in Christ" and one translation expressed the phrase, "in union with Christ". That's why sex is not just a sport or a casual human behavior of pleasure or even procreation; it expresses the intimacy of a person's relationship with God through Christ. This is precisely Jesus' central message of John 15 in which He declared that He was the vine and the believer the branch that is grafted into a living union with the vine.

Sarah Young has beautifully and sensitively captured this reality.

> I am Christ in you, the *hope of Glory*. The One who walks beside you, holding you by your hand, is the same One who lives within you. This is a deep unfathomable mystery. You and I are intertwined in an intimacy involving every fiber of your being. The Light of My Presence shines within you, as well as upon you. I am in you, and you are in Me; therefore, nothing in heaven or on earth can separate you from Me!

> As you sit quietly in My Presence, your awareness of My Life within you is heightened. This produces the Joy of the Lord, which is your strength. I the God of hope, fill you with all Joy and Peace as you trust in Me, so that you may bubble over with hope by the power of the Holy

Spirit. (Colossians 1:27; Isaiah 42:6; Nehemiah 8:10; Romans 15:23 (AMP).[42]

Having explored the theological implications of the metaphor, how does this approach contrast with the prevalent viewpoints on sex in today's culture? What are the moral implications in an orgasmic sex-driven society? Is situation ethics a viable viewpoint?

---

42   Sarah Young, *Jesus Calling: Enjoying Peace in His Presence* (Nashville, Tennessee: Thomas Nelson, 2004), 332.

Sex expresses the spiritual union of two who are not seeking to get something, but to bring fulfillment to each other, both equally giving and equally receiving. Coercing another to prove their "love" by having sex is only animal lust—a hunger we are trying to fill.

7

IS SEX PURELY A PERSONAL CHOICE?

I detect today a certain public skepticism when intellectuals stand up to preach to us, a growing tendency among ordinary people to dispute the right of academics, writers and philosophers, eminent though they may be, to tell us how to behave and conduct our affairs.... A dozen people picked at random on the street are at least as likely to offer sensible views on moral and political matters as a cross-section of the intelligentsia (Paul Johnson).[43]

"Dear Ann Landers: They buried my lover today. We were 'together' for 25 years. I had no part in the funeral and no grieving with anyone except a friend in whom I confided.

I am married to a man I respect but do not love. My lover felt the same way about his wife. We stayed with our mates because of our families. My grief is deep, and my loss is beyond words. My life was a secret, and now my pain must be secret also. Guilt and pain are a terrible exchange for a few stolen moments.

---

43   Johnson 342.

> Whatever relationship you have with your wife or husband, work at it, stick with it and get help if you need it, but don't get involved with a married person.
>
> Fortunately for me, our secret died with him. Now I need to forgive myself. Tell your readers to remain faithful. I wish I had (N.Y., July 9, 1993)."

Any discussion of sex must include a discussion of morality, especially if integrity and commitments are emphasized. Trust must have a moral standard agreed upon by both parties or it cannot exist. If I say I love someone, and that means to me a commitment to care for, appreciate, respect, and give to that other person, but they view love as a narcissistic means to fill their own hungers, I will end up hurt and deeply distrustful of the other. Bruce Kaye, in a discussion of "Foundations for Morality,"[44] pointed out that situation ethics brought an emphasis upon love as the ultimate criterion for making a decision, rather than one being bound by a code of some sort. That sounds noble, but it can become too subjective and hence undermine the absolutes stated in Scripture. How love is defined, and how a person applies it in a given situation is critically important. The Bible's definition centers in a unique word, *agapē* (pronounced, agap'-ay), the Greek word for God's kind of love, stands sharply contrasted eroti nd even friendship love in its selflessness. C.S. Lewis described *agapē* as not a hunger that needs to be filled, but a fullness that gives away.[45]

---

44   See Robin Keely, ed., *Eerdmans' Handbook to Christian Belief* (Grand Rapids, Michigan: Wm B. Eerdmans Publishing Co., 1982), 287 for a more complete discussion.

45   A taped radio broadcast in a Word records tape the author no longer has in his possession.

Paul Johnson examined the lives of Jean-Jacques Rousseau, Shelley, Karl Marx, Henrik Ibsen, Bertrand Russell, Jean-Paul Sartre and others. He describes their pursuit of hedonistic pleasure and addiction to sensual pleasure in sexual exploits, drugs, and multiple marriages or affairs. The result was the discarding of their children and the abuse of the women with whom they sought to satisfy their lust.

The Bible's point is that if we truly loved another person, we would limit our sexual involvement to the security of a long-term, committed relationship. Its essence is to bind itself to another, not to float free, jumping from one lily-pad to another like a frog hoping for an encounter that will suddenly make it a prince. The "prince" has integrity in which his word has meaning. He has dignity and worth found in a personal relationship with God and he doesn't look for promiscuous sex to bring the longed-for intimacy. Sex, instead, expresses the spiritual union of two who are not seeking to get something, but to bring fulfillment to each other, both equally giving and equally receiving. Coercing another to prove their "love" by having sex is only animal lust—a hunger we are trying to fill. We get our word, "erotic," from the Greek word, *eros*. If humans actually loved with God's love, it would be an adequate determinant of decisions. But our love is polluted by a sinful nature that finds more attraction to lust. *Agapē* only comes through the intimacy of "knowing" God. Through His union with the human spirit it is possible for lust to be transformed into love and a biblical sexual morality attained.

A simple comparison of television sitcoms of the fifties
and sixties with today's sitcoms demonstrates that cultural
mores have become explicit and sometimes crude. What has
brought about the change? John and Paul Feinberg wrote: "The
value system of any culture lends structure and organization
to it, and a major element in any culture's value system is its
understanding of human sexuality.... The decade between
1945 and 1955 saw the traditional consensus on sexuality
erode. The Sexual Revolution began in this period. Monogamy
was not universally praised; penicillin and the pill removed
three of the most undesirable consequences of promiscuity:
infection, detection and conception."[46] They identified six
factors contributing to the changes that have taken place. First
was the acceptance of secularism as a dominant worldview.
"This is the view that God must be removed from all areas
of human thought and activity."[47] Second was privatization.
"It is commonly held that many areas of life, especially one's
sexual preferences, are one's own business."[48] Third was what
they termed scientific frankness. "This meant that any attempt
to limit sexual expression is psychologically harmful, and
even capable of making one insane." Fourth, media exposure
began to permeate lives in subliminal ways with a "constant
bombardment of depersonalized, seductive sex." A fifth
factor was existential schizophrenia. "Reality and personal
meaning have been divorced. The real is what is scientifically
quantifiable and verifiable. Emotions such as love and purpose

---

46   John S. Feinberg and Paul D. Feinberg, *Ethics for a Brave New World*
(Wheaton, Illinois: Crossway Books, 1993), 150.

47   *Ibid.*

48   *Ibid.*, 151.

are not quantifiable. Therefore, they are not real, but they have personal meaning. What results is a distinction between values and behavior." Sixth and last, therapeutic values: "Values that govern the counselor in his or her work are becoming the values of society as a whole. The counselor must be accepting, sympathetic and understanding if the client is to be helped."[49]

The question is often asked, what would Jesus do? He was a full-blood male. Did He have sexual desires and drives? Some novelists have exploited that theme but are they on target?

What Would Jesus Do?

Another approach proposed to making moral decisions is to seek to follow Jesus' model. Thomas à Kempis' *The Imitation of Christ* was built upon this premise as was a more contemporary approach in Sheldon's *In His Steps*. The problem with the "What would Jesus do?" question, is the natural tendency to subjective interpretation. In addition, Jesus did not marry, and there isn't a shred of historic evidence to suggest he had any sexual encounters with women, notwithstanding the films, "The Last Temptation of Christ" or "The da Vinci Code". How then can a person ask, "What would Jesus do?" What is the Jesus model of sex? It would not conflict with the Old Testament's clearly defined sexual morality. He would not participate in pre-marital sex, adultery, homosexuality, bestiality, and other non-heterosexual marital sex.

Perhaps a more provocative question is why did Jesus not marry? If God created sex and the marriage bed is pure

---

49   *Ibid.*

(Hebrews 13:5), surely it would not have been sinful for him as man to marry and thus participate in conjugal love. His uniqueness as the God-man and His role as Savior precluded marriage and fathering children. What would His wife have become through the union? What would His children have been—themselves God and human? That is preposterous. His celibacy does not lower sexuality. It rather strongly affirms self-control and abstinence for young men and women. He, too, knew the dynamics of sexuality. This raises the question of Jesus' own struggle with lust—did he?

Jesus was a human male—every bit as human as any man—but with one difference. He was not born with the crippling and distorting sinful nature that is more attracted to darkness than light. Jesus said we love darkness rather than light because our deeds are evil. We run from light. Did he do so, too? No. He was light and His light repels darkness. As a result, Jesus could relate to women at a different level without the insidious desire to mentally strip them or view them as objects of sexual conquest. Can other men ever get to that level? Maybe not with perfection, but we can surely do better than most have so far! How is that possible? The powerful principle stated by Paul of the mystery of the Gospel—Christ in you the hope of glory! Jesus living in us by the Holy Spirit will empower us to live a life of sexual constraint and control.

Why is there a seeming dramatic difference in the subject of sex in the Old Testament and what we read in the New Testament?

The Sexy Old Testament and the Non-Sexy New Testament

To today's reader the Old Testament is crammed full of sex and the New Testament is almost non-sexual. Why is this? Paul declared in Christ there is neither male nor female. Jesus delivered Mary Magdalene, a profligate woman, from the demons that drove her. He rescued a woman caught in adultery from the jeering accusations of religious leaders. But there isn't a David and Bathsheba, or a Judah's visit to what he assumed was a prostitute. None of the disciples had a Hosea-type experience though they proclaimed God's Word to sinful people.

Christ raised marriage from law to love by His imparted grace. Paul did not say, husbands love the brethren as you love your wife. He said love your wife as Christ loved the church. In Christ the Spirit writes on our hearts first; then we bring our behavior into conformity to the transformed heart.

The church in the first three centuries wrestled with the question of the deity of Jesus that resulted in the Council of Nicaea's statement on the Trinity. It was also concerned about the dominating, powerful drive of sex and how is it to be properly understood. Respected Princeton scholar, Peter Brown summarized the history of the church fathers in *The Body and Society*. His account of early father, Tertullian, demonstrates the church's attempts to establish an appropriate understanding of sex. "Renunciation and baptism into the Church declared the power of sex null and void. Possession of the Holy Spirit conferred by baptism was thought to lift men and women

above the vast 'shame' of the human condition."[50] Joining
in attitude with secular society was a misogynous attitude
about women. "The misogyny to which Tertullian appealed
so insistently was, in his opinion, based on unalterable facts
of nature: women were seductive, and Christian baptism did
nothing to change this fact."[51] The Church had to face the
reality of the irrefutable place of sex in society. "Sexuality was
based on a drive that was widely spoken of as irresistible—a
current Greek euphemism for the penis was 'The Necessity.'
This drive, furthermore, was the known cause of the one
irrefutably unidirectional process to which human beings freely
contributed—procreation."[52]

In the early years of the twenty-first century, it is obvious
that western civilization is adrift without a commonly accepted
definition of moral and sexual standards. David Neff wrote
of the controversy of family values that ricocheted around
the country in the 1992 presidential election. "Honesty,
dependability, self-control, and having a clean conscience were
once *virtues*; then they became *values*; and now, apparently,
they are *prejudices*."[53] Neff argued that Americans have lost
any hope for some unified moral vision. Conscience is not
adequate, for there is no generally acceptable source to inform
the conscience. Any subjective approach that leaves the
individual to judge for their self is flawed unless that person

---

50   Peter Brown, *The Body and Society: Men, Women, and Sexual Renunciation in Early Christianity* (New York: Columbia University Press, 1988), 80.

51   *Ibid.*, 81.

52   *Ibid.*, 84.

53   David Neff, "American Babel," *Christianity Today*, 17 August 1992, 18.

has a plumb-line against which to measure the action. For the Christian, the Bible is that plumb-line.

Another factor that has produced a lack of an accepted sexual code has been identifiable shifts in how people see life and sexual experience as a part of life. Lewis Smedes listed four. First, the Enlightenment brought a focus on the individual so that sex exists to meet personal needs. Perhaps it needs to be pointed out that humans have been promiscuous throughout history as is evidenced by the Canaanites and Ninevites of the Bible. However, Smedes focused on the shift in morals in Western Civilization and the United States. As a result, there no longer is a shared purpose for human life.

Second, with God reduced from the God of the Bible to a generic term only—god with a small "g"—came a loss of authority. The individual and the scientific community are the only authorities that are recognized. Further, all authority is distrusted and the loss of sexual moral authority is a reflection of that fact.

Third, there has been a loss of morality itself. "Where there are no moral imperatives but only strong tastes, judgments about what is good or bad in sexual conduct are eroded. If you happen to like the homosexual lifestyle, enjoy your own thing; but don't judge homosexual people. If you are offended by such things as extra-marital flings, group sex, or pornography, cultivate your own feelings; but don't condemn others."[54]

---

54   Lewis B. Smedes, "The Changing Sexual Scene," Robin Keeley, ed., *Christianity in Today's World* (Grand Rapids, Michigan: Wm B. Eerdmans Publishing Co., 1985), 353.

Values Clarification in public education attempted to reduce morality to a student's subjective how-do-you-feel-about-it. It seems this is the only way to approach morality when God is no longer allowed voice in a classroom. Morality requires a religious base, and religion has been shut out of the classroom. Morality needs a measure that is external to humanity. Culture has moved from an external moral standard to an internal moral norm. This subjective norm is not consistent and cannot be applied to others. It's my thing. For society to function without chaos, requires an objective norm that is enforced by law. The internal norm is totally inadequate due to a predisposition to sin.

The fourth shift, says Smedes, is a loss of sense of mystery. By the cognitive/ laboratory approach to understanding the sex act, we have erased the mystery that is an inherent part of the God who created sexual people in His own image. "Christians believe that there is the symbolic meaning and the reality of a deep personal union to which we have given the name of marriage. For this reason, sex can be symbolic of the union between Jesus Christ and the church. This mystique has always been a buttress for the traditional sexual morality; anything signifying so deep spiritual reality must be kept in its proper place and for its proper purpose."[55]

The love of Christ for the church is symbolic of marital love that includes sex. That is quite different than sex being symbolic of the union of Christ and the church. It is also a far cry from the Los Angeles sex-based Church of the Most High Goddess. The wife/priestess claimed to have had sex with over

---

55   *Ibid.*, 354.

1,000 men in a two year period with the promise of salvation for those who indulged. Their claim was that their church ought to be protected as a religion, rather than she prosecuted as a prostitute. The deepest spiritual significance in sex lies in the metaphor in which the LORD comes to "know" His people. That turns the marriage bedroom into a temple and it becomes an act of worship, as is eating and working and playing, in celebrating the love and joy of a saving God.

The shifts identified by Smedes are 180 degrees out of phase with the character of a God who has entered into a commitment with His people. If marriages enjoyed the security of integrity and commitment, suspicion would not undermine the relationship producing hostility, nagging, coldness and sometimes violence. People building faith together brings security and builds confidence. As couples build the integrity of a marriage, that integrity forms a boundary against infidelity. United in the strong bond of marital integrity, a couple enters a level of intimacy that moves them into a likeness to God. Without integrity, relationships disintegrate. Through the promises of God the believer actually shares in the divine nature so that he or she can escape the moral disintegration in which the world is trapped (2 Peter 1:3-4, J.B. Philipps). God's promises depend upon His integrity to keep His word, and our sharing in His nature means we can participate in His integrity and therefore possess a power to live within God's boundaries. God's saving grace makes it possible for the believer to participate in relationships built upon unfailing love, compassion, and faithfulness. Only through "knowing" God in this intimate way can people be rescued from their

own inner depraved drives, and from the moral morass into
which the western world has sunk. Jesus described the intimacy
of believers with Him in the same language of His intimacy
with the Father: "On that day you will realize that I am in my
Father, and that you are in me, and I am in you" (John 14:20).
Paul wrote along the same lines: "He who unites himself with
the Lord is one with him in spirit" (1 Corinthians 6:17). The
biblical phrase, "in Christ" can be rendered, "in union with
Christ." The sexual metaphor portrays the characteristics
that make a life of relationships work, and nowhere more
effectively than in a loving, sexual marriage of a woman and a
man.

God has placed His Church in this shifting moral scene
to be a point of constancy for His moral standards. However,
the church hasn't been there for the most part. There hasn't
been any input on the spiritual and theological core of sex.
Unanswered questions have resulted in one of the most
powerful drives in a man or woman going unchecked. The
church's failure to explain God's parable has made sex a
playground of the devil. Not only that, celibacy in one branch
of Christianity has generated some of the greatest sex scandals
to ever undermine the church as a moral authority. The moral
failure of prominent evangelical pastors and leaders has echoed
the scandalous Elmer Gantry.

All of God's controlling statements are purposeful. The
biblical relationship of husband and wife fosters the best
environment for healthy sex. The church has only addressed the
surface issues of "just say no" because of disease and babies.

We can do better. God expects us to and it centers on who he is. The question is how.

Why They Waited Until They Married[56]

In a recent video and accompanying story published by fashion and beauty website Refinery29, the outlet covers Gunnar and Sarah Larson, a couple who made the decision to remain abstinent — one that isn't generally given a great deal of attention these days. While neither was a virgin at the time of their engagement, the two were brought up in religious homes and decided to exercise their faith by waiting for one another.

Described as a "hopeless romantic," Larson told Refinery29 that he actually bought his wife's engagement ring when he was only 13 years old — nearly 10 years before he met Sarah, and that ring ended up fitting her perfectly.

"We had our first date, our first kiss and — we didn't have sex," Larson explained, recounting the couple's love story. "We both kind of came from a religious background. We were saving ourselves for marriage. The funny thing is neither of us technically saved ourself for marriage."

But Larson, a New York City-based interior designer, said that their relationship afforded them a renewed opportunity to do just that.

"We felt like we could kind of redeem ourselves and give this gift of our sexuality to each other," he said.

Larson went on to share details about their wedding night, describing their first time as a "spiritual moment" of coming together.

56   http://www.theblaze.com/stories/2015/02/12/why-this-couple-decided-to-wait-until-marriage-to-have-sex-and-the-message-this-dad-wants-his-daughter-to-learn-about-love/, (Accessed 2/23/2015).

He also said that he wants his own daughter, whom he and his wife had five years into their marriage, to know "true love" and that he believes he and Sarah have something special.

"Our love and our footprint of who we are together builds us - like makes us stronger," he said.

If a person understands the true spiritual nature of sex, they will be more willing to respect and implement the disciplines of delayed gratification and confinement of sex to the covenanted marital relationship of a man and woman.

8

THE BOTTOM LINE
(SO TO SPEAK)

*"How can a young person stay pure? By obeying your word....
I have hidden your word in my heart, that I might not sin
against you"* (Psalm 119:9, 11 NLT).

*"And I am certain that God, who began the good work within
you, will continue his work until it is finally finished on the
day when Christ Jesus returns.* (Philippians 1:6 NLT).

Hormones bouncing all over the body. Eyes unable to avoid
the seductive messages of skin-tight clothing and generously
exposed cleavage, media advertising that sells sex rather than
the product, TV shows, movies, a scantily-clothed pop singer's
soft porn, MTV, magazines, newspapers, and even bumper
stickers seek to entice to immoral thoughts and action. Ears are
bombarded with explicitly sexual lyrics. Delaying marriage
until an education is gained and a career with income secured.
It all combines to say, "No way. I can't counter it all. God is
out of touch. It may have worked in those days, but, like, hey,
that was 3,000 years ago. A little outmoded." It is good to seek

to be financially stable when entering marriage, but no career or amount of money is of greater importance than integrity. Memories can haunt people. When you are with your spouse, former partners are going to be in the room—even in the bed. That's not what you want to happen! To answer the question of how a person can follow what appears in our culture to be an impossible standard we need to establish some basic assumptions about sex.

First, God made sex. It was not the result of something called "Random Chance." Who is "Random Chance" but an expression about mathematical possibilities? Sex is good. When God finished His creative work, He said it was good. The notion that biblical Christianity is anti-sex is groundless. It is true that various aspects of institutional Christianity have been out of kilter, but the Bible says sex is good.

Second, the purpose of sex is to bring unity and pleasure to the participants as well as to procreate the species. God is not against pleasure. He is the One who made sex the powerful and enjoyable thing it is. In the beginning, God spoke of a couple being joined together as "one flesh" (Genesis 2:24). The underlying unity is spiritual, which is expressed physically. God made us first as spiritual beings. The spirit is the key to meaning and that, in turn, to satisfaction and fulfillment. God works from the spirit to the flesh. That is why sex as sport inevitably bankrupts the spirit. It denies the essential personhood of the individual. Sexual intercourse is to assist the development of the spiritual oneness of the married couple as both partners enjoy the physical fulfillment of orgasm, and are "welded together" in purpose, goal, desire, love, and commitment. To omit the latter is to leave one hollow. Such can happen within marriage, but is inevitable in promiscuity.

A third assumption is the Bible knows what it's talking about and is an infallible guide to human behavior. The problem is not with the Bible, it is with humans who interpret it and who are subject to their own sinful preferences. Human beings are born with a handicap of sin that hinders understanding and biases behavior. It is only through the saving grace of God in Jesus of Nazareth, and the Holy Spirit's living within the human heart that behavior can be conformed to the will of a holy God. But it can be done. Ideas are powerful and do shape behavior. Ideas listened to by people today state, "Do it. It's great. Don't stay within the lines." God's ideas are also powerful. They must be spoken with relevance and enthusiasm, and those who submit will find they are right and they work. At best, however, people understand and behave with limited perfection.

A concluding assumption: Those who accept the parameters of Scripture, by faith allow the Holy Spirit to give them personal inner strength and choose to obey God by staying within His lines will receive superb rewards. What are the benefits for doing it God's way? How can I stay within the boundaries? We'll address biblical answers in the next chapter, but first, God speaks.

Leviticus 18 Sex[57]

God spoke to Moses, "Speak to the People of Israel. Tell them: I am God, your God. Don't live like the people of Egypt where you used to live, and don't live like the people of Canaan where I'm bringing you. Don't do what they do. Obey my laws and live by my decrees. I am your God. Keep my decrees and laws: The person who obeys them lives by them. I am God.

Don't have sex with a close relative. I am God.

Don't violate your father by having sex with your mother. She is your mother. Don't have sex with her.

Don't have sex with your father's wife. That violates your father.

Don't have sex with your sister, whether she's your father's daughter or your mother's, whether she was born in the same house or elsewhere.

Don't have sex with your son's daughter or your daughter's daughter. That would violate your own body.

Don't have sex with the daughter of your father's wife born to your father. She is your sister.

Don't have sex with your father's sister; she is your aunt, closely related to your father.

Don't have sex with your mother's sister; she is your aunt, closely related to your mother.

Don't violate your father's brother, your uncle, by having sex with his wife. She is your aunt.

Don't have sex with your daughter-in-law. She is your son's wife; don't have sex with her.

Don't have sex with your brother's wife; that would violate your brother.

---

57   Eugene H. Peterson, *The Message: The Bible In Contemporary Language* (Omaha, Nebraska: QUICKVERSE, A Division of Findex.com, INC.)

Don't have sex with both a woman and her daughter. And don't have sex with her granddaughters either. They are her close relatives. That is wicked.

Don't marry your wife's sister as a rival wife and have sex with her while your wife is living.

Don't have sex with a woman during the time of her menstrual period when she is unclean. "Don't have sex with your neighbor's wife and violate yourself
by her.

Don't give any of your children to be burned in sacrifice to the god Molech—an act of sheer blasphemy of your God. I am God.

Don't have sex with a man as one does with a woman. That is abhorrent.

Don't have sex with an animal and violate yourself by it. "A woman must not have sex with an animal. That is perverse.

Don't pollute yourself in any of these ways. This is how the nations became polluted, the ones that I am going to drive out of the land before you.

Even the land itself became polluted and I punished it for its iniquities—the land vomited up its inhabitants. You must keep my decrees and laws—natives and foreigners both. You must not do any of these abhorrent things. The people who lived in this land before you arrived did all these things and polluted the land. And if you pollute it, the land will vomit you up just as it vomited up the nations that preceded you.

Those who do any of these abhorrent things will be cut off from their people. Keep to what I tell you; don't engage in any of the abhorrent acts that were practiced before you came. Don't pollute yourselves with them. I am God, *your* God."

I was bound by the iron chain of my own will. The enemy held fast my will, and had made of it a chain, and had bound me tight with it. For out of the perverse will came lust, and the service of lust ended in habit, and habit, not resisted, became necessity. By these links, as it were, forged together--which is why I called it "a chain"—a hard bondage held me in slavery. But that new will which had begun to spring up in me freely to worship thee and to enjoy thee, O my God, the only certain Joy, was not able as yet to overcome my former willfulness, made strong by long indulgence. Thus my two wills--the old and the new, the carnal and the spiritual—were in conflict within me; and by their discord they tore my soul apart.... For the law of sin is the tyranny of habit, by which the mind is drawn and held, even against its will. Yet it deserves to be so held because it so willingly falls into the habit.[58]

---

58   Augustine's *Confessions*: Book 8, chapter 5

9

HOW TO KEEP THE DRIVE WITHIN GOD'S BOUNDARIES

No test or temptation that comes your way is beyond the course of what others have had to face. All you need to remember is that God will never let you down; he'll never let you be pushed past your limit; he'll always be there to help you come through it (1 Corinthians 10:13, The Message).

No temptation has overtaken you but such as is common to man; and God is faithful, who will not allow you to be tempted beyond what you are able, but with the temptation will provide the way of escape also, so that you will be able to endure it (1 Corinthians 10:13, NASB).

Dear friends, you always followed my instructions when I was with you. And now that I am away, it is even more important. Work hard to show the results of your salvation, obeying God with deep reverence and fear. For God is working in you giving you the desire and the power to do what pleases him (Philippians 2:12-13, NLT).

I was in the eighth grade in a Christian school. We were asked to choose a life verse. Like most teens, I was coming alive to sex and found it a huge area of test. I am very grateful for a Christian family that had instilled a respect for God and biblical morality, so I chose this verse as a life verse:

"No temptation has seized you except what is common to man. And God is faithful; he will not let you be tempted beyond what you can bear. But when you are tempted, he will also provide a way out so that you can stand up under it" (1 Corinthians 10:13).

Little did I understand at that time that it would be a lodestar for decades to come not only regarding sex, but many other areas of testing and temptation. We need the Holy Spirit beside us as our *Paraclete* (John 14) at every stage of life, not necessarily in the same category of sex, but relationships, anger, greed, career choices, power and money.

The Bible not only outlines God's standards and principles related to human behavior, it also addresses how redeemed, yet sinful, people can alter ingrained patterns. Here are some primary biblical principles:

- A person is forgiven and cleansed from sin through the redemption that is in Christ (Ephesians 1:7).

- A person is given divine life (regenerated) by the Holy Spirit uniting with the human spirit and making her or him a new creation (Titus 3:4-7; 1 Corinthians 6:17; 2 Corinthians 5:17).

- The Holy Spirit is available and desirous to take control of the mind, emotions and will to establish new values, transform our desires and motivate our wills to choose to obey God's commands (Galatians 5:22-25). He does not force His mastery and so enslave a person. Rather He waits to be invited to carry out His ministry of conforming the person to Jesus (Ephesians 5:18; Romans 8:5). Conformity to Jesus is a life of true love, God's kind of love, for He is love. Love is not something that He gives away; it is who He is as a person. The only way people can love at His level is to have Him living in them in controlling power by His Spirit.

- The process of becoming like Jesus is lifelong and includes a struggle (battle) of the flesh against the Spirit (Galatians 5:17). Let's take a closer look at these spiritual dynamics.

We must begin with love. Henry Drummond, author of the classic *The Greatest Thing in the World*, wrote that love is the *summum bonum*—the supreme good. He wrote at the close of the eighteenth century, Drummond, a scientist and not a clergyman or academic, discussed the love chapter of 1 Corinthians 13. Drummond examined the nine characteristics as stated by Paul as a prism breaking love into multifaceted colors of beauty, love is seen in its behavior: patient, kind, generous, humble, courteous, unselfish, of good temper, guileless, and sincere.[59] Paul used the special word, *agapē* (ἀγάπη) for love. As previously identified, agapē is not a hunger that needs to be filled, but a fullness that gives away. Love of this quality will not ask a girlfriend to "prove" her love by having sex. It will not look at sex as simply a sport, a fling or "doing what comes naturally." Eros is the word for lust. *Agapē* is far more complex and virtuous. Greek scholar, William Barclay, wrote: "*Agapē* has to do with the mind: it is not simply an emotion which rises unbidden in our hearts; it is a principle by which we deliberately live. *Agapē* has supremely to do with the will. It is conquest, a victory, an achievement.

---

59   Henry Drummond, *The Greatest Thing in the World* (Westwood, New Jersey: Fleming H. Revell Company, no date), 136, 24.

No one ever naturally loved his enemies. To love one's enemies is a conquest of all our natural inclinations and emotions. This *agapē,* this Christian love, is not merely an emotional experience which comes to us unbidden and unsought; it is a deliberate principle of the mind, and a deliberate conquest and achievement of the will."[60]

> In the Christian tradition love (especially *agapē*) is an expression of the essential nature of God, the perfect characterization of the relationship between God and humans, and the supernatural virtue or character of God reflected in the Christian community in relation to God and one another as shaped by the indwelling Holy Spirit. This connection between love and God's own character gives rise to the Christian focus on love as the fundamental characteristic of Christian discipleship and hence of Christian ethics. Many Christian thinkers suggest that the essence of love is unconditional giving of oneself for the sake of others.[61]

John, the loving apostle, boldly stated that "God is love." He did not say God has love as though it was something separate from Himself that He could give to another. The only way to have the love of God in one's life is to have God Himself living, motivating, and enabling one to love as He loves. Drummond argued that what makes love the *summum bonum*—the supreme good—is that it lasts when everything else is finished, including faith and hope. "To love abundantly is to live abundantly, and to love forever is to live forever.

---

60   William Barclay, *More New Testament Words* (New York: Harper & Brothers Publishers,1958), 15.

61   Stanley J. Grenz, David Guretzki, Cherith Fee Nordling, *Pocket Dictionary of Theological Terms* (Copyright © 1999. All rights reserved, Electronic Edition STEP Files Copyright © 2007, QuickVerse. All rights reserved).

Hence, eternal life is inextricably bound up with love. We want to live forever for the same reason that we want to live tomorrow. Why do we want to live tomorrow? Is it because there is someone who loves you, and whom you want to see tomorrow, and be with, and love them back? There is no other reason why we should live on than that we love and are beloved." His summary statement is "eternal life is to know God, and God is love." As powerful as that is, Drummond concluded his argument that when we stand in judgment we will not be asked what we believed, but did we love. The rest of religion, the final test of religion, is not religiousness, but love, not what I have done, or believed, or achieved but how I loved.[62] The unique heart of Christianity is a life of love, which is not a result of following religious rules or ritual, but the supernatural power of the Holy Spirit, the Spirit of Jesus, living in us and producing His fruit: love (Galatians 5:22-23).

This is a challenge. To track Paul's rationale, we need to clarify the terms he uses. In Romans 6:6 he stated the "old self was crucified with him (Christ), so that the body of sin might be done away with, that we should no longer be slaves to sin." The word translated "old self" (NIV), is the word, *anthropos*, or man, the translation used in the King James Version. John Stott, in his book, *Men Made New*, brought the concept into focus. He observed our existence as Christians is broken into two volumes. Volume one begins with our natural birth. In that natural state there is a built-in aversion and resistance to God that causes us to choose sin over righteousness from our earliest discernment. Our default response is sin. When we

---

62   Drummond, 49-63.

come to Christ the natural state comes to an end in death—we are crucified with Christ. Because of that fact, the controlling power of sin is broken creating a new "default" response ability to obey God.

However, there is a carryover of the old self into the new self. This Paul calls the "flesh". By this, he does not mean our physical flesh, but a spiritual dynamic of the pre-conversion life that is 180° out of phase with God. This dynamic is always present, never fully goes away and is the source of the internal battle.

A person is more than a physical being, a composite of chemicals. Therefore, science alone will never be able to fully answer the question of human behavior. Since we are spiritual in the core of our being, we need to understand the spiritual dynamics at work in shaping and motivating behavior.

When Paul confronted the Judaizers by categorically denying the role of the Law in achieving a right relationship to God, he had to then face the question of the origin and control of behavior. He emphatically stated it is not by Law, *i.e.*, attempting to keep a moral code of some sort. That is not to say society should not have law to protect its citizens. It is to say that law (religious or civil) is incapable of solving the problem of wrong behavior. Law or rules of behavior are only effective to the degree they control behavior, but totally incapable of changing the heart from which behavior derives. I will illustrate this in a later chapter relating to church law.

For example, prohibition did not stop Americans from making or drinking alcohol. Anti-abortion legislation will not stop abortion. Women will seek doctors who perform abortions. Law does not change a person's motivation. It does help to control anti-social behavior or in the case of abortion the destruction of helpless innocent human life. The real issue is the heart.

The reason Law (meaning God's Law as stated in the Ten Commandments, the moral law) is unable to solve the problem is that it represents the spiritual standard of a holy God as applied to people who are spiritually dead and therefore incapable of responding. A person must receive spiritual life through a personal union with God. This (called regeneration) occurs when God the Holy Spirit is fused with the human spirit. When a person repents of their sinful condition and places their trust in Jesus Christ as Lord and Savior they are united with the Holy Spirit. As the Holy Spirit takes up residence within the heart, He begins to motivate and direct behavior enabling one to keep God's standard of righteousness. It is a radical change, so much so that Paul said if a person is in Christ she or he is a new creation (2 Corinthians 5:17). It is God's work of grace in the human heart. God always initiates the action. The human responds to God's activity in agreement, trust and obedience.

Paul's critics said: "If you destroy Law people will be released to live abandoned lives of sin." His answer was:

- Sin is a product of an internal force called the sinful nature, or the flesh.

- The sinful nature is ours by birth.

- The resolution to this problem is the Holy Spirit

bringing the very life and nature of God to our hearts to counteract our sinful nature.

Galatians 5:16-18 outlines two forces within us locked in conflict. It portrays the sinful nature battling the Spirit. What is the "sinful nature"?

The sinful nature defined: an inherited force within every human being that causes us to behave in sinful ways. It runs throughout the whole of our spiritual system causing us to malfunction. It is not some separate entity that can be excised by spiritual surgery. "Desire" refers to the sinful nature having a strong driving compulsion.

At the same time the Holy Spirit "desires" what is contrary to the sinful nature. Who is the Spirit? He is the Holy Spirit, the third person of the Trinity; He is God who personally lives in the believer beginning at conversion. When a person trusts in Christ, she or he is regenerated. That includes the whole of life being infused by the presence of the Holy Spirit. The Holy Spirit does not live in a compartment of our life, but rather permeates our whole being.

"The real truth is that when the Holy Spirit regenerated me, He regenerated *me*. He did not merely transfer to me, or create inside me, a new 'nature'; He infused new spiritual life into and throughout *my own human nature* so that I became a spiritually renewed human being. And having been thus regenerated, I myself, in my own human nature, may become more and more refined by that same gracious Holy Spirit...." [63]

---

63   J. Sidlow Baxter, *A New Call to Holiness* (Grand Rapids, MI, Zondervan Publishing House, 1973), 32.

The Spirit is Himself a strong, driving compulsion within the believer. Romans 6:12-13 is emphatic: "Do not let sin control the way you live, do not give into sinful desires. Do not let any part of your body become an instrument of evil to serve sin." Notice the verb "let" is used twice. It communicates that the human being is not boxed in to be a slave of his or her appetites. The apostle spoke from experience. He knew the full thrust of various physical drives and had wrestled with them. He found a source of power adequate to equip him to live in freedom and purity.

The Flesh/Spirit Conflict Prevents Desired Behavior

Galatians 5:17: "They are in conflict with each other so that you do not do what you want."

Romans 7:21: "So I find this law at work: When I want to do good, evil is right there with me."

Romans 7:18: "For I have a desire to do what is good, but I cannot carry it out."

Our problem is not a lack of knowledge of right and wrong, but of the power to do the right. The power is ours in the person of the Holy Spirit who literally lives in the believer, joined to her spirit. With best intentions and prayer, we will not eliminate the inner conflict instituted by the flesh warring against the Spirit until we are finally released into the direct presence of God. In a devotional discussion of this passage in Romans 7, James Packer wrote: "In reality, it is a mark of spiritual health passionately to desire to be perfect for the glory of God and then to be deeply distressed when one finds that sin, though dethroned and no longer dominant, remains within, marauding and trying to regain control, so that one cannot fully achieve righteousness. This healthy distress at the way in which, morally speaking , what one aims for always exceeds what one actually grasps is what Romans 7:24-25 portrays."[64]

The Sinful Nature's Behavior Described
(Galatians 5:19-21; 1 Corinthians 5-6; Ephesians 4:17-31))

Paul wrote to believers describing the dynamic of our daily experience. The Christian is not only capable of these behaviors; we do them because we have a sinful nature. These behaviors are not simply mistakes, bad judgment, or a moment of weakness, which they certainly are. These behaviors are sins and must be dealt with as such. We read in Galatians 5:19: "The acts of the sinful nature (*sarx*: flesh) are obvious: sexual immorality, impurity and debauchery; idolatry and witchcraft; hatred, discord, jealousy, fits of rage, selfish ambition, dissensions, factions and envy; drunkenness, orgies and the like." The first sins in the list are sexual sins.

- **Sexual immorality** (*porneia*), any immoral sexual relationship--immoral as defined by biblical statements. *Porneu* was used of prostitution, to pay another for sexual favors. It isn't limited to sex for pay, but having sex with anyone other than one's husband or wife.

- **Impurity** (*akatharsia*), described the idea of being dirty and applied particularly to language and the mind: a dirty mouth or dirty mind. Telling dirty stories and listening to them is of the flesh.

- **Debauchery** (*aselgeia*), refers to a full lack of self-control, total self-indulgence, the absence of restraint.

---

64   James Packer, *Your Father Loves You: Daily Insights for Knowing God*, compiled and edited by Jean Watson (Wheaton, Illinois: Harold Shaw Publisher,1986), March 21.

Excessive, compulsive masturbation, drunkenness (whether alcohol or other drugs), overeating or turning to food as a source of personal comfort, or laziness are illustrations.

With that brief summary, let's address our primary concern: how a Christian can live within the boundaries of God's plan for sex. How can the dynamic drive that is a healthy expression of God-given sexual experience be harnessed and limited to God's boundaries rather than scribbling all over the page in sexual indulgence?

The following bullet points state the actions God expects us to take. He has done His part. Now we are to do ours.

- Come to the Lord Jesus Christ as a sinner; place your full trust in Him alone to forgive you, come into your life and transform you from the inside out. When you cross that threshold you will become a new creation where the old is gone and the new has come. This is God's work inside you. It is a required point of beginning. Without it, God cannot empower you to live a righteous life.

- The majority of believers stop there. A second threshold needs to be crossed. It can occur at the same time as the first, but it is not the same transaction. Most come to a realization at a later time in their Christian experience that there is a dual authority: Jesus and self. The conflict can be significant and the frustration over repeated failure intense. Step two requires total, voluntary submission to the Holy Spirit to live the life of Jesus in us.

Romans 12:1-2 challenges the person who has established a right relationship with God (Romans 1-5) and is experiencing the frustration of Romans 7, to present their bodies as a living sacrifice to God. A useful term for this is full surrender of one's entire life to the Lord. At this stage a person realizes that living the slogan "it's all about me" has not produced the longed for quality of life. The person of the Trinity that seeks a body to live in and through is the Holy Spirit. Although the Spirit takes up residency in the believer at conversion, He now has freedom to express His authority and power in every area of life. When the Spirit rules and the believer obeys, frustration is replaced by satisfaction and righteousness replaces sin and rebellion. As Galatians 5:22-23 reads: "The fruit of the Spirit is love, joy, peace, patience, kindness, faithfulness, gentleness and self-control."

In the same way that Jesus does not invade a person's life but gently knocks at the door of the heart asking to come in, the Holy Spirit does not fill or take control of a life until invited to do so. God respects the personal choice of His creation. However, although there is a specific time in stepping across the threshold of request, this is not a one-time choice but must be a conscious moment by moment, daily reality.

It would certainly be ideal if the above resulted in a flawless life. That isn't the case. 2 Peter 3:18 states we are to "grow in the grace and knowledge of our Lord and Savior Jesus Christ." In similar language, Paul challenged us to "keep in step with the Spirit" (Galatians 5::25). This is not an impossible achievement, since the real victory was won by Jesus on the cross when he conquered sin. Paul wrote that those who belong to Jesus "have crucified the sinful nature (flesh) with its passions and desires" (Galatians 5:24-25). The original grammar is helpful in understanding this statement.

It is in the perfect tense. "The perfect tense suggests that Paul
is thinking of that specific completed event which marked
his identification with Christ and which has had an enduring
effect upon his life."[65] Paul was like any other man and faced
sexual fantasies and persistent urges, yet he found strength and
resolve in Jesus' indwelling presence. He wrote the Corinthians
that since our bodies are the habitation of the Holy Spirit and
members of Christ Himself (1 Corinthians 6:13-20), we are
to not have sex with prostitutes or with anyone other than
our spouse. The phrase translated into English as "sexual
immorality" in the NIV is *porneia* (πορνεία). A narrow use of
the word applies to prostitution, but the general application
is extramarital intercourse. [66] Paul flatly declared that "the
body is not meant for sexual immorality (*porneia*), but for the
Lord." He boldly challenges the believer to "flee from sexual
immorality. All other sins a man commits are outside his body,
but he who sins sexually sins against his own body" (:18). Our
bodies don't belong to us, they belong to Christ who bought
and paid for them with His blood. Sex is not all about "me".
For the Christian, it is all about Jesus who is the Master, having
bought us at a terrible cost on the cross.

In 1 Corinthians 7:9 when discussing sexual ethics for the
formerly married, Paul addresses the role of self-control. There
the word is *egkrateuomai* (ἐγκρατεύομαι) or self-restraint.
To give clarity to the concept of self-control over physical

65   Fritz Rienecker and Cleon Rogers, *Linguistic Key to the Greek New Testament* (Grand Rapids, MI: Regency Reference Library, 1980), 507.
66   Gerhard Kittel and Gerhard Friedrich, ed., translated by Geoffrey W. Bromiley Abridged by Geoffrey W. Bromiley, *Theological Dictionary of the New Testament* (Grand Rapids, Mich.: William B. Eerdmans Publishing Company. 1985), Electronic Edition STEP Files Copyright © 2007, Findex.Com. All rights reserved.

drives and impulses, Paul used the same expression in 9:25. Using the metaphor of competition in athletics, the athlete will exert enormous discipline to get in shape to win a race. The same word appears, *egkrateuomai*, only translated in the NIV as "strict training." In that passage Paul stated the level and cost of the discipline in the Christian life. This is no easy matter. It takes far more self-leadership than a simple prayer. The root from which *egkrateuomai* is taken refers to power, dominion, strength or government. The phrase self-leadership applies. This is rigorous training to the point that Paul said, "I beat my body and make it my slave." The original language is beat one's face black and blue (ὑπωπιάζω, *hupōpiazō*)[67]. Obviously this is not to be taken literally but metaphorically to describe the challenge. That is extreme sport discipline, only in the Christian life it is not a temporary trophy, but an eternal reward. Psychologists consider this type of behavior as delayed gratification. The challenge is to delay sex until marriage.

How is this done? Where does a testosterone driven teen or twenty male to get the internal resources to pull this one off? The New Testament is very clear; it is by the power of the Holy Spirit who has been connected to the human spirit to empower one to live a God-pleasing life sexually.

When Paul stated a "mind set on what the Spirit desires," he expressed that a believer is to focus on God and not on the flesh or the sinful nature with the behaviors listed in Galatians 5. This is not an easy task assuming the God-given drive of

---

67   Note Thayer: to beat black and blue, to smite so as to cause bruises and livid spots 1a) like a boxer one buffets his body, handle it roughly, discipline by hardships.

sex coupled with the powerful influence of the various media bombarding our minds with sexual images and invitations.
A person is responsible to control what they read, look at, or listen to. God isn't going to do that for us. We choose every moment of every day what activities we will engage in. The Spirit will inwardly warn us when we are about to choose the wrong direction, but the choice remains ours. To visit porn sites on line or buy skin magazines that feed sexual urges will not promote restraint. Because of the inherent power of the sex drive and our default inclination to immoral thought and action, our aggressive prayer must be: "Jesus, this is bigger than me. I can't win this; you must win the battle of impulsive lust. I put my sex drive on the cross for you to crucify all that is impure and set free all that is pure and in line with your purposes." Of course there is forgiveness in the grace of a loving Father when we fail and as often as we repent and turn from our disobedience and sin (1 John 1:9).

As we grow in the above spiritual life skills, we will reap life-long benefits. Perhaps a little time spent in a personal study will reinforce the concepts we have outlined to this point. I invite you to take ten to twenty minutes for the next few days to delve into God's Word. After you go through the following inductive study on spiritual transformation based on 2 Peter 1, we'll look at the benefits of living within the boundaries, consequences of disregarding the boundaries, and conclude our discussion by looking at the failure of the church historically to understand or appropriately address the issue of sex.

A Personal Study Guide toward Spiritual Transformation and Coping with the Sex Drive

- Right thinking precedes right behavior.

- Right thinking begins with the mind understanding and accepting God's Word as true.

"For all of God's promises have been fulfilled in Christ with a resounding 'Yes!' And through Christ, our 'Amen' (which means 'Yes') ascends to God for his glory" (2 Corinthians 1:20 NLT)

- **Theme:** Developing a Harmonious Life

- **Scripture:** 2 Peter 1:3-11

- **Task:** Determine specific areas of character development needed to become spiritually whole based on the virtues of growth outlined by Peter.

Verses 3-4–primary statements:

"By his divine power, God has given us everything we need for living a godly life. We have received all of this by coming to know him, the one who called us to himself by means of his marvelous glory and excellence. And because of his glory and excellence, he has given us great and precious promises. These are the promises that enable you to share his divine nature and escape the world's corruption caused by human desires" (NLT).

- God has given everything we need for life and godliness

- God has called us to such a life

- It is ours through an intimate knowledge of God, which He has given us through great and precious promises

- These promises are the means to intimacy, i.e., participation in the divine nature

- As the divine nature controls us, we escape the corruption that is in the world through lust (desires that demand immediate gratification contrary to God's intended fulfillment); J. B. Phillips translation: "making it possible for you to escape the *inevitable disintegration that lust produces* in the world and to share in God's essential nature." [Italics the author's for emphasis.]

This passage is another biblical affirmation that God is the one who changes the heart. Out of a changed heart comes changed behavior. Theories of behavior modification and the role of law in a society have a limited capacity to alter behavior. Humanity is fallen, broken, and needs a Savior. Only in Jesus is there an offer of regeneration: *"If anyone is in Christ he is a new creation; the old has gone, the new has come"* (2 Corinthians 5:17). That is why Jesus told a religious and good man he had to be born again, not only to get into heaven, but also to have a new heart.

What is a promise? "They are words said or written, binding a person to do or not to do something."

What are some promises that give life and power? Write a summary phrase of the promise:

- 1 Corinthians 2:12
- 1 Corinthians 10:13
- 2 Corinthians 2:14-16
- 2 Corinthians 9:8
- Philippians 1:6
- Philippians 2:12-13
- Philippians 4:12-13

- 1 Peter 1:3-4
- 2 Timothy 1:7
- James 1:5
- Psalm 32:8

Where are promises found?

- Numbers 23:19
- Joshua 23:14
- Romans 4:20-21
- Jeremiah 15:16
- Psalm 119:9, 11, 50, 58, 162

How does a promise become a source of personal transformation?

- Knowledge: a person cannot personalize a promise from God if he or she doesn't know it exists
- Personal need: a promise might be known, but will lie dormant until a need arises that triggers access to the promise
- Faith: appropriate or personally take the promise

Why do this hard work?

Without it we will remain infantile Christians and will be subject to the disintegrating lusts that pound us into ruin.

> Romans 12:2 "Don't copy the behavior and customs of this world, but let God transform you into a new person by changing the way you think Then you will know what God wants you to do, and you will know how good and pleasing and perfect his will really is" (NLT).

Seven Character Qualities in Christian Spiritual Formation that Grow out of Faith

Paul wrote to the Philippians (3:8-11):

What is more, I consider everything a loss compared to the surpassing greatness of knowing Christ Jesus my Lord, for whose sake I have lost all things. I consider them rubbish, that I may gain Christ and be found in him, not having a righteousness of my own that comes from the law, but that which is through faith in Christ—the righteousness that comes from God and is by faith. I want to know Christ and the power of his resurrection and the fellowship of sharing in his sufferings, becoming like him in his death, and so, somehow, to attain to the resurrection from the dead.

Peter informs us that the knowledge of Christ provides us with everything we need for life and godliness and then outlines **how** we can develop a life of godly character. The divine nature becomes dynamic within the believer through personal faith appropriation of God's promises. God gives new life, but character is not an automatic result. I have to develop it. God works in us to help us want to do His will and give the power to do it, but we make the behavioral choices each day. Godliness (*eusēbeia*) is "the attitude which gives God the place he ought to occupy in life and in thought and in devotion…. (It) gives God the *right place*, and worships God in the *right way*."[68]. This word is listed as one of the virtues to be developed by the believer.

Emotional maturity requires a unified self, as one scholar expressed it. That occurs when everything is oriented around

68   William Barclay, *More New Testament Words* (New York: Harper & Brothers, 1958), 68.

one goal. Jesus said in Matthew 6:33 that we are to seek first God's kingdom and righteousness and then the rest of life will fall into place. In 1 Thessalonians 5:24 Paul prays that our whole spirit and soul and body be kept blameless. If a unified self is seen in this concept it might look something like this:

- Spirit: fellowship with God, sensitivity to others, creativity (new birth, submission to Christ as Lord)

- Soul: emotions, intellect, volition (will)

- Body: physical needs, clothing, food, housing

To integrate the self around the central purpose of Christ and His righteousness will result in wholeness. To focus part of self on someone or something other than Christ will open us to disintegration. That is the core of the battle of the flesh verses the Spirit.

The English word for "holy'" is of Anglo-Saxon derivation meaning "well, or whole". In James 1:4 the result of perseverance in the tests of life is that we can become "mature and complete, not lacking anything." Maturity expresses itself in a right relationship with God: to love God with all "your heart and with all your soul and with all your mind". It also requires a right relationship with people: "love your neighbor as yourself". [Matthew 22:37-39].

Because of these facts of what God has done, Peter states the believer's responsibility. It begins with attitude and focus of energy: "Make every effort." Barclay translated this section: "Bend all your energy to the task of equipping your faith with…."

"Equipping" refers to the word, *epichorēgein*. At its root it refers to the leader of a chorus. Because the chorus in Greek drama was central to the great celebrations, it was very costly to recruit and train the participants. "The word, therefore, has a certain lavishness in it. It never means to equip in any cheese-paring and miserly way; it means lavishly and willingly to pour out everything that is necessary for a noble performance."[69]

A number of years ago I asked our grandson, Jack, to mow our lawn and edge it while we were gone for a couple of weeks. At that time he was in early junior high. His Dad told me when I returned of his discussion about how poorly Jack had done his work the first week. "I wouldn't ask you back if that's how you did my lawn. You do good work and Pops will hire you again." After he finished the second time, being careful to get all the grass and trim it correctly, he said, "Dad that really looks good."

When we make every effort to apply ourselves to develop these qualities, we will also have the sense of "that was good." Personal worth, a healthy self-image, is a product of living a godly life.

2 Peter 1:5-7:

In view of all this, make every effort to respond to God's promises. Supplement your faith with a generous provision of moral excellence, and moral excellence with knowledge, and knowledge with self-control, and self-control with patient endurance, and patient endurance with godliness, and godliness with brotherly affection, and brotherly affection with love for everyone (NLT).

---

69   William Barclay, *The Letters of James and Peter* (Philadelphia: The Westminster Press, 1958), 352, 353.

There are seven character qualities identified, each of which grows out of faith, that is like the tap root of a plant, and the preceding quality: moral excellence grows out of faith, knowledge grows out of faith and moral excellence, self-control grows out of faith and knowledge, patient endurance grows out of faith and self-control, godliness grows out of faith and patient endurance, brotherly affection grows out of faith and godliness, love grows out of faith and brotherly affection. Vincent commented the phrase 'add to' means to "develop one virtue in the exercise of another…an increase by growth not by external junction; each new grace springing out of attempting, and perfecting another."

Faith (*pistis*) is defined as 'firm conviction'. This is the soil in which the flower of virtues grows. It is the tap root of a plant. If the tap root gets chopped, the plant or tree will die. The reason the Bible has been attacked throughout the centuries is because faith comes by hearing the Word of God. Our firm conviction is that the God of the Bible is the only God; the Bible is His revelation to humankind; and that He is the author of the manual on life and His way is the right way to live. Faith is firmly convinced that obedience has the joyous result of God's blessing and disobedience also brings consequences, only the ones we don't want. Faith is based upon the Word of God, and therefore the more I know God's Word, the stronger my faith will become.

Hebrews 11:1-6: "The bed seed of faith is the conviction that what matters most is more than matter…. The faithful believe God exists, and he rewards those who pursue him."[70]

Summarize the place of the Bible and the ministry of the Holy Spirit in the following verses:

- 2 Peter 1:1, where does faith come from?
- James 2:14-26, explore the relation of faith to action.
- John 15, branches in living union with the vine will produce fruit. What role does faith play?
- Zechariah 4:6 states the role of the Holy Spirit in the development of faith and spiritual power. How is that power accessed?

Who gives the Holy Spirit and how is he received? Luke 11:13

Peter states the role of the Spirit in spiritual growth. State each verse in a bullet point: 1 Peter 3:18; 1:2 1:10-12;
2 Peter 1:21.

A basic faith issue is the reliability of the Bible. Ours is an age of religious and spiritual deception. Without a thorough working knowledge of the Bible, we will not have the firm conviction to keep us on track when confronted with convincing and logical alternatives.

Years ago Scotland Yard conducted a private exhibition of forged paintings for art dealers. The objective was to send a warning to their select audience about the sale of forgeries, which some experts estimate make up forty percent of the art market.

---

70   Mark Buchanan, *Hidden in Plain Sight: the Secret of More* (Nashville, TN: Thomas Nelson, Inc., 2007) 29.

The forgeries at the exhibit were created with remarkable proficiency. Reliance on documentation alone won't solve the problem because even that is often forged! Fiona Ford, of the Association of Arts & Antiques Dealers, said the level of skill displayed by the forgers was "terrifying." She added, "If every dealer saw this exhibition, it would further impress on them how careful they have to be."[71]

Goodness (*arētē*): moral excellence. It is the virtue that makes a person good. Moral excellence is the ability to discern right and wrong as expressed by the holiness of a righteous and pure God. Spiritual discernment must penetrate the moral relevancy of a secular humanistic philosophical system. It is the compass for the believer in a perverse and morally dislocated culture. We are in an age of moral blindness. The only reliable source of informing our conscience is the Word of God. Moral excellence grows out of knowledge of the Word, the source of faith.

Moses' experience of God's goodness: Exodus 33:19; 34:5-7

Peter's experience of God's goodness: Matthew 3:17. In 2 Peter 1:16-18 the glory of God is His goodness.

How to develop moral excellence (goodness):

- Become a true worshipper (1 Peter 2:9)

- Walk in the Spirit (Galatians 5:22-25; 2 Corinthians 3:17-18). Be ruthless with sinful attitudes and behaviors. Quickly confess and repent of sin (1 John 1:9).

---

71   Associated Press, "Police Display Fakes at Exhibition to Warn Art Dealers," www.topix.net (posted on 11-23-06).

- Imitate good people (3 John 1:11)[72]

Knowledge (*gnōsis*): practical knowledge of what to do, how to live life. Proverbs is a manual on how to live life. "*Gnosis* is that knowledge which enables a man to decide rightly and to act honorably and efficiently in the day to day circumstances and situations of life."[73] In secular Greek, *gnōsis* refers to knowledge gained by experience. It is widely used in New Testament to refer to Gnosticism. "The New Testament writers frequently found themselves in conflict with travelling preachers who had their own version of the apostolic *kērygma*. Timothy was expressly warned against the 'godless chatter' and the 'contradictions' of knowledge (*gnosis*) falsely so called (1 Tim. 6:20)."[74]

Epignōsis: "It has, however, quite clearly an intellectual, semi-dogmatic stress. The knowledge of God's truth is of equal importance with experiential profession of the Lord, and finally pushes it into the background. Hence, conversion to the Christian faith can be described almost technically as coming to a knowledge (*epignōsis*) of the truth (1 Tim. 2:4; 2 Tim. 3:7; cf. Heb. 10:26; 1 Tim. 5:3; 2 Tim. 2:25; Tit. 1:1; 2 Pet. 2:21)."[75]

Give a bullet point summary of each of the following passages:

- Job 38:18-19; 39:1

- 1 Corinthians 8:1

- 2 Peter 1:2*, 3*, 5, 8*; 2:1-3 [false teachers]; 2:20*

---

72   See Buchanan, 4-85.
73   Ibid., 357.
74   Colin Brown, General Editor, *Dictionary of New Testament Theology* (Grand Rapids, MI: Zondervan Publishing House, 1971), Vol. 2, 405.
75   Ibid., 405.

Epignōsis: fullness of understanding or complete understanding that comes piece by piece in a lifelong process. "The stronger term *epignōsis* is used to denote the full and more perfect knowledge which is possessed in Christ, the conditions of which are humility and love."[76]

- Colossians 2:2-3

- Peter was a fisherman, not a trained scholar (Acts 4:13). What did observers say was his and the other apostles' source of boldness?

- Ephesians 1:17* How does this prayer of Paul express the above reality?

Self-control (*egkrateia*): Self-discipline is the battle of the Holy Spirit against unbridled lust that never ends, but that enables a person to grow in victory. Passion remains, but it is under control, not out of control. Christians are not passionless robots. It is a key in the non-stop battle of the flesh versus the Spirit; without it, we will never be able to stand against the wiles of a clever enemy whose one goal is our spiritual destruction.

Summarize Peter's expression for the need of spiritual power: 1 Peter 1:13-16; 4:17; 5:8; (note Peter's failure: Matthew 16:22 with Luke 22:31-32, 34)

Areas of Self-Control:

- Time

- Talents, personal gifting

- Thought life

---

76   *International Standard Bible Encyclopedia,* "Know, Knowledge," Electronic Edition STEP Files Copyright © 1998, Parsons Technology, Inc., all rights reserved.

- Entertainment
- Tongue
- Money

Perseverance (*hupomonē*): "It is the quality which keeps a man on his feet with his face to the wind. It is the virtue which can transmute the hardest trial into glory because beyond the pain it sees the goal. It is the spirit which can bear things, not simply with resignation, but with blazing hope."[77]

Summarize Peter's expression of this quality:

1 Peter 1:10-11; 5:1;

2 Peter 1:11; 3:11b-13

John was on the same page with Peter. He emphasized the need to stay the course because there is no other option: John 6:68-69

Value of suffering:

Refines faith: 1 Peter 6-7

Perfects hope: 1 Peter 1:8-9; 1:21

Weans from sin: 1 Peter 4:1-3

Deepens intimacy with Jesus: 1 Peter 4:12-13

Trains in holiness: 1 Peter 4:16-19

Peter buckled under the pressure of friends: Galatians 2:11-14 (this was after his encounter with the other apostles in Acts11 when he defended his going to the home of Cornelius).

What do these passages teach about perseverance?

---

77   William Barclay, *A New Testament Wordbook* (New York: Harper & Brothers, no date), 60.

- Romans 5:3-5
- Hebrew 2:10; 5:8-9
- Isaiah 43:1-2
- Psalm 9:9; 16:1; 18:2; 34:8; 36:7; 46:1; 71:1 (refuge)
- Psalm 28:7; 59:17; 73:26; 96:7 (strength)

Wrong responses to adversity result in stress (see Holmes-Rahe stress test conclusions about the effects of stress).

Right responses:

- Accept that God loves you and has allowed adversity to come for good reasons
- Thank him for the very thing that is the source of stress because he will give shelter and strength
- Declare him to be your refuge and strength
- Face only today's problems; don't borrow from tomorrow or live under the cloud of yesterday

Godliness (*eusēbeia*): "The man who has *eusēbeia* always correctly worships God, and gives God His due; but the man who has *eusēbeia* always correctly serves his fellow-men, and also gives men their due…the man who is in a right relationship both with God and his fellow-men."[78]

> The root meaning of *eusēbeia* "is awe in the presence of that which is more than human, reverence in the presence of that which is majestic and divine; …a worship which befits that awe, and a life of active obedience which befits that reverence. The fact is that in so far as Greek has a word for region that word is *eusēbeia*."[79]

---

78   Barclay, *Letters of Peter*, 358-359.
79   Barclay, *More NT Words*, 67.

Adversity is the soil for developing godliness. It is learning to see life, including adversity, from His perspective. Not only are we to persevere in adversity but to seek to grasp what God is doing in us or through us in that circumstance.

True worship, then, requires obedience to how God asks us to respond to adversity. We are to be doers of the word and not hearers only. Worship is more than being emotionally moved by music or enjoying a sermon skillfully crafted and delivered.

- 1 Peter 1:16, what is the Old Testament reference and how does a person "obey" this command?
- 1 Peter 3:15, why is the quality of our behavior so critical to the task of telling the good news of the gospel?

"If Godliness is God-centeredness, worldliness is self-centeredness. It's craving, lusting, boasting. It's me, me, me…. Worldliness is whatever makes sin look more attractive than God."[80]

Briefly summarize the themes of these verses. What are you asked to do; why are we told to take this action; or, what does God say he will do or provide?

- 1 John 2:15-17
- Colossians 3:1-3; Hebrews 12:12-13
- James 4:7-10

There are three expressions of godliness in 1 Timothy:

- 1 Timothy 3:16: "the mystery of godliness" is that Jesus is God come in the flesh. He is the exclusive way to God.

---

80   Buchanan, 155.

- 1 Timothy 4:7-8: "Take time and trouble to keep yourself spiritually fit. Bodily fitness has a certain value, but spiritual fitness is essential, both for this present life and for the life to come. There is no doubt about this at all, and Christians should remember it" (J. B. Phillips, *The New Testament in Modern English*).

- 1 Timothy 6:3-11: (3-5) godliness is the evidence of sound teaching; (6-8) "godliness with contentment is great gain"; (9-10) "the love of money is a root of all kinds of evil" and demonstrates money is a greater value than godliness.

- 2 Timothy 3:12: "Everyone who wants to live a godly life in Christ Jesus will be persecuted."

- 2 Peter 3:11: "Since everything will be destroyed in this way, what kind of people ought you to be? You ought to live holy and godly lives as you look forward to the day of God and speed its coming."

The New Testament depicts the ethical as the supreme and permanent work of the Spirit. Paul begins his survey of the ideal life by characteristic references to its redemptive foundation, and he repeatedly concludes his practical exhortation to godly living with a reference to the power of the Spirit.... The Risen Christ gives to humanity a new moral power. That power is Christ himself, by the Spirit, as the inward energy of the moral life which flows from regenerate human nature.[81]

Brotherly kindness (*philadelphia*): means love of the brethren. This applies even to enemies: "You have heard it said, 'Love your neighbor and hate your enemy.' But I tell you: Love

---

81   Carl F. H. Henry, *Christian Personal Ethics* (Grand Rapids, MI: Wm B. Eerdmans Publishing Co, 1957) 440, 443.

your enemies and pray for those who persecute you" (Matthew 5:44).

Summarize the following verses on brotherly love:

- Romans 12:10

- 1 Thessalonians 4:9

- Hebrews 13:1

- 1 Peter 1:22, note two different Greek words are used for love; why do you think Peter did this?

- 1 Peter 3:8

Certain ants in South and Central American rainforests will lie down in the potholes that stand between their army and food. Their bodies form a makeshift bridge, allowing other ants—sometimes numbering over 200,000—to make better time in getting to the source of nourishment.

This pattern in the life of ants was discovered through research done at England's University of Bristol. Researchers took a wooden plank and drilled different sized holes in it, simulating a narrow trail. Ants would find holes equal to their size and lay down inside, letting others walk safely over them. When the raiding party accomplished its mission and was returning to its nest, the faithful few climbed out of their holes and followed the raiders home.

Love (*agapē*): Not a hunger that needs to be fed, but a fullness that gives away. "While the Hebrew and Greek words for 'love' have various shades and intensities of meaning, they may be summed up in some such definition as this: Love, whether used of God or man, is an earnest and anxious desire for and an active and beneficent interest in the well-being of the one loved."[82]

- Matthew 5:43-48

- John 13:34-35 (*agapē*); 15:10-13, 17

- How is God's love for us a model of how we are to love one another? Romans 5:6-10

- 1 Thessalonians 4:9 "…you have been taught by God to love one another" (*agapaō*)

- Romans 12:9-10; "Love (*agapē*) must be sincere…. Be devoted to one another in brotherly love (*philadelphia*)."

- Romans 13:10 "Love (*agapē*) does no harm to its neighbor. Therefore love is the fulfillment of the law."

- 1 Peter 2:17

- 1 John 3:10-18; 4:7-21

- Peter's challenge: John 21:16

"It [*agapē*, love] wills to love even in the face of fierce resistance…. It's an in-spite of love….It is unprovoked love"[83]

> The more you grow like this, the more productive and useful you will be in your knowledge of our Lord Jesus Christ. But those who fail to develop in this way are shortsighted or blind, forgetting that they have been cleansed from their old sins. So, dear brothers and sisters,ᵉ work hard to prove that you really are among those God has called and chosen. Do these things, and you will never fall away. Then God will give you a grand

---

82   "Agape, James Orr, General Ed., *International Standard Bible Encyclopedia* Electronic Edition STEP Files Copyright © 1998, Parsons Technology, Inc., all rights reserved.

83   Buchanan, 179.

entrance into the eternal Kingdom of our Lord and Savior Jesus Christ (NLT).

Having spent some time in inductive study, let's pick up where we left off in our discussion of the sex metaphor. I had concluded that following God's directives about sex would produce gratifying benefits. What are they?

But, wretched youth that I was—supremely wretched even in the very outset of my youth—I had entreated chastity of thee and had prayed, 'Grant me chastity and continence, but not yet.' For I was afraid lest thou shouldst hear me too soon, and too soon cure me of my disease of lust which I desired to have satisfied rather than extinguished. [84]

I was saying these things and weeping in the most bitter contrition of my heart, when suddenly I heard the voice of a boy or a girl I know not which--coming from the neighboring house, chanting over and over again, 'Pick it up, read it; pick it up, read it'.... I could not but think that this was a divine command to open the Bible and read the first passage I should light upon.... I snatched it up, opened it, and in silence read the paragraph on which my eyes first fell: "Not in rioting and drunkenness, not in chambering and wantonness, not in strife and envying, but put on the Lord Jesus Christ, and make no provision for the flesh to fulfill the lusts thereof." I wanted to read no further, nor did I need to. For instantly, as the sentence ended, there was infused in my heart something like the light of full certainty and all the gloom of doubt vanished away. [85]

---

84   Augustine's *Confessions*: Book 8, Chapter 7.
85   Ibid., Chapter 12.

ex is to be used to serve our spouse, as well as the analogy that our restlessness for the sexual experience mirrors our restlessness for God.... God made flesh, and when God made flesh, he created some amazing sensations. While the male sexual organ has multiple functions, the female clitoris has just one—sexual pleasure. By design, God created a bodily organ that has no other purpose than to provide women with sexual ecstasy. This wasn't Satan's idea—it was God's. And God called every bit of his creation 'very good'" (Genesis 1:31). [86]

---

86   Gary Thomas: *Sacred Marriage: What if God designed marriage to make us holy more than to make us happy?* (Grand Rapids, Michigan: Zondervan, 2000), 201,206-207.

10

A Satisfying Life-Long Relationship

It is beautiful to see a couple still in love after fifty or more years of marriage. Most people born after 1950 won't have a shot at that long-term enjoyment because they've been through several marriages. They will grow old. They may have a partner. But they won't have the same person who shared all the same memories of the children, vacations, travel, entertainment events, and the scrap-book of good times and hard times.

It is ironic that God created male and female—sex—to answer the loneliness of man's condition in the beginning. Through the fall of humankind in sin, sex was cursed with loneliness and shame. The first thing Adam and Eve did was to look for some type of covering for their nakedness.[87] Why is it that what was designed by God to express the deepest level of intimacy of which the human is capable, can result in emptiness and loneliness when it is outside of lines, or abused because of selfishness coming from a heart driven by lust?

87   See Jones for a more complete theological discussion.

It is because the spiritual dimension of sex demands that its expression stay within the lines of a heterosexual monogamous marriage, preferably with people who have experienced God's saving grace making them new persons. Keeping inside the boundaries will also prevent soul destruction. It will increase one's sense of worth.

Increased Personal Worth

There is an abundance of evidence that our sense of personal worth is associated with our adherence to a standard of ethical and moral behavior. If a person can control the expression of one of the most powerful drives in the human body, it can greatly increase a sense of worth and achievement. Peter wrote that we are to *"abstain from sinful desires, which war against your soul"* (1 Peter 2:11). The soul to the Greek was the center of emotions. Sin wars against emotional health. No sin damages self-worth more than sexual sin because it concerns an essential nature of God. It's about character, integrity, faithfulness, trust—the primary stuff that makes up a good life. Could anything cut more deeply than to be negatively compared to someone else's sexual performance? Promiscuity sets up a person for hurt. God has placed the boundaries of sex within marriage to provide the protection of faithfulness, trust, and acceptance.

In the summer of 1956 the Westmont Quartet—a public relations male quartet of which I was a member—was guest of Youth for Christ in its annual youth conference at Winona Lake, Indiana attended by some 5,000 teens. Billy Graham, who launched his evangelistic career in that organization, was the featured speaker. In his sermon he stated no sin sears the conscience more quickly than sexual sin. Sex is a central factor in human experience, spiritually and psychologically.

A person's identity should not be based on performance whether that is in business, athletics, the arts, or in bed. A Christian is loved and accepted by God on the basis of their relationship with Christ. Performance contributes to self-worth but is only one part of the mix. There is likely to be someone better; a world record will eventually be broken. Age or illness will take away the ability to perform. In Christ, every person is fully accepted, appreciated, and loved, totally apart from performance—even spiritual performance. Because of the unconditional love and acceptance a person has in Christ, they do not have to look to anyone else, or any other relationship to give them value. They are of value because God has bound Himself to them in a covenant of unfailing love. As Paul expressed it so dramatically, nothing can *"separate us from the love of God that is in Christ Jesus our Lord"* (Romans 8:37-39). In Christ a person enjoys full personal security.

Personal Security

Can you trust your spouse when he or she isn't with you? Can you give him or her freedom to enjoy other friendships, or are you always suspicious of something going on that will spark a new interest? Why do people have these feelings? The soaps and sit-coms focus on fooling around giving the message that it is the norm for society. If partners have had their flings, what will prevent the same thing happening again if some difficulties are encountered in the marriage? Keeping sex within the lines of marriage frees from suspicion and the nagging it generates. It gives security and the freedom to respond to one's spouse with enjoyment.

Those are some of the benefits of sexual restraint. God is not only the source of love. He is also just. Justice demands a consequence for the violation of His moral standards. While we might be uncomfortable in today's politically correct cocoon, God is the only being in the universe that holds in perfect balance, love and mercy with justice and judgment. What does God's judgment look like?

We are free to choose certain behaviors; we are not free to choose the consequences of those actions.

11

FACING THE REALITY OF JUDGMENT

"Thus says the LORD: 'Stand by the roads, and look, and ask for the ancient paths, where the good way is; and walk in it, and find rest for your souls.' But they said, 'We will not walk in it.'" (Jeremiah 6:16 ESV)

"If you know God, you know He is absolutely and perfectly just. But we have to define this term first. What do we mean by justice? In looking this up very carefully in the Scriptures, I find that justice is indistinguishable from righteousness in the Old Testament. It's the same root word with variations according to the part of speech used. It means uprightness or rectitude. To say that God is just or that the justice of God is a fact is to say that there is uprightness and rectitude in God.... Justice and righteousness are indistinguishable from each other....

"The word 'judgment'... is the application of justice to a moral situation, favorable or unfavorable. When God judges a man He brings justice to that man's life. He applies justice to the moral situation which that man's life created. And if the man's ways are equal, then justice favors the man. If man's ways are unequal then, of course, God sentences the man.

"Justice is not something that God has. Justice is something that God is. A grammarian might say it should be phrased, 'Just is something that God is.' But I say, "No, justice is something that God is." God is love and just as God is love, God is justice."[88]

It may not be the most popular subject in the tabloids, among students, or adults, but it is a reality. A severe punishment was established in the Hebrew culture for adultery. The God of the Hebrews hasn't changed. He is the same God in the New Testament. Ancient Mosaic laws called for the stoning of people caught in adultery. Not because God is a tyrant, but Moses repeated the need for discipline within the community to *"purge the evil from among you."* Betrayal and the lack of integrity as expressed in adultery are evil and will destroy a civilization. Violating sexual ethics leads to other immoral behaviors. It powerfully mars the distinguishing of right from wrong.

"In order of us to fully experience the freedom of God, we must be fully free to do both good and evil. God's 'punishment' establishes value. It is not vindictive. It is a consequence of our behavior, the same as my touching a hot stove. The consequence is getting burned. There is the judgment of nature and the judgment of God's wrath against sin nationally and personally."

88   A.W. Tozer, *The Attributes of God: A Journey into the Father's Heart* (Camp Hill, PA: Christian Publications, Inc., 1997), chapter 4, QuickVerse e-publication.

Nature's Judgment

The judgment of disease crosses all boundaries of age, status, race, culture, government, education, wealth or poverty. Why sexually transmitted diseases (STD's)? Why the acquired immune deficiency syndrome (AIDS)? People who steal don't get diseases from doing so. People, who gossip, tell lies, slander another's character, cheat on exams, even murder, don't get diseases from doing so. Nature has put limits on sex. If there had never been sexual promiscuity, if there had only been heterosexual, monogamous marriages throughout the ages and now, there wouldn't be any of these horrible, wasting diseases. Why the judgment? Because nature itself is screaming at us that sex is sacred. It is not a sport. People are not to fool around. Thankfully, modern medicine has developed antibiotics that take care of most STD's. Instead of controlling sexual behavior, people have only used it as license to fool around more.

Studies have suggested that teen sex is linked to depression and suicide tries. *USA Today* reported that "about 14% of girls who have had intercourse have attempted suicide; 5% of sexually inactive girls have. About 6% of sexually active boys have tried suicide; less than 1% of sexually inactive boys have. Tamara Kreinin of the Sexuality Information and Education Council of the United States stated, 'We need to take depression among the young very seriously.' But it is a 'disservice' to blame sexual activity and ignore 'divorce, domestic violence, sexual abuse, substance abuse, lack of parental and community support and questions about sexual orientation,' she said."[89]

Abortion is mostly a method of birth control used by unmarried women (over 90%) who for a variety of reasons have chosen to not marry, and to enter into sexual relationships but not employ adequate birth control methods. Given that the fetus is human life, abortion is a judgment of death by the mother on the baby because of the mother's sexual behavior. Is there a parallel of a mother's sentence of death upon her child in abortion to the death sentence of the ancient Hebrew people upon adulterous partners? The one dying in abortion is totally innocent and undeserving of death.

National Judgment

"How can I pardon you? Your children have forsaken me and have sworn by those who are no gods. When I fed them to the full, they committed adultery and trooped to the houses of whores. They were well-fed, lusty stallions, each neighing for his neighbor's wife. Shall I not punish them for these things?' declares the LORD; 'and shall I not avenge myself on a nation such as this?" (Jeremiah 5:7-9 ESV)

Adultery, or sexual immorality, is a metaphor of betraying God. This is why severe judgment is attached to it. After having recited the various terms of God's covenant that included specific guidelines for sexual behavior, Moses warned of the consequences of Israel's breaking the covenant. God said: "*I am making this covenant, with its oath, not only with you who are standing here with us today in the presence of the* LORD *your God but also with those who are not here today*"

89   *USA Today*, June 4, 2003, 8D.

(Deuteronomy 29:14)—meaning the generations to come. The language of Moses demonstrated he knew the people would fail. After the calamities of the curses listed in Deuteronomy had occurred, people would ask, *"Why has the* LORD *done this to this land? Why this fierce, burning anger? And the answer will be: 'It is because this people abandoned the covenant of the* LORD, *the God of their fathers, the covenant he made with them when he brought them out of Egypt"* (29:24-25).

What kind of judgment did God forecast would come for turning from him and impudently defy the lines He established for sexual expression? He said he would *"strike you with wasting disease, with fever and inflammation, with scorching heat and drought, with blight and mildew, which will plague you until you perish"* (28:22). Other forms of judgment included military defeat, the carnage of war that would include women raped, wives taken and personal property plundered, and finally captivity in a foreign land. All of those curses came upon Israel and Judah in time. Not a pretty picture!

The church at the beginning of the twenty-first century has shied away from the severity of God's wrath against sin in an effort to avoid criticism and make the gospel more palatable. Yet, even an elementary reading makes clear He is a God of judgment as well as tender mercy and loving grace. For what reason would God spare the United States or any other contemporary country from these curses given the life-style and defiance of biblical morality prevalent around the world? What is the correlation of world-wide tragedy and governmental dysfunction with the breakdown of sexual morality? We are free to choose certain behaviors; we are not free to choose the consequences of those actions. God has established the law of cause and effect; we are not able to change it.

The Personal Judgment of Hell

> But as for the cowardly, the faithless, the detestable,
> as for murderers, the sexually immoral, sorcerers,
> idolaters, and all liars, their portion will be in the lake
> that burns with fire and sulfur, which is the second death
> (Revelation 21:8 ESV).

As horrible as these national judgments were, there is something far worse for the individual, and that is God's judgment in hell. Paul warned the morally liberal Christians in Corinth that certain people would not be in heaven. "*Do not be deceived: Neither the sexually immoral nor idolaters nor adulterers nor male prostitutes nor homosexual offenders nor thieves nor the greedy nor drunkards nor slanderers nor swindlers will inherit the kingdom of God*" (1 Corinthians 6:10). He clarified that it did not mean there was no hope for people who had been guilty of those sins, for he went on to say, "*And that is what some of you were. But you were washed, you were sanctified, you were justified in the name of the Lord Jesus Christ and by the Spirit of our God*" (11). The gospel is that God forgives, cleanses the inner life, and makes a person new in condition and standing before God. Therefore, the argument runs, people's behaviors are to change when they come to Christ. If the behavior doesn't change, it is likely the person has never received the new heart that God gives in Christ. An adulterer or promiscuous person can get a second start through Christ. God totally forgives and wipes the slate clean, but only in and through Christ. A person with a new heart has a new start. They are not to continue in the old behavior patterns. The last book of the Bible warned that the sexually immoral, along with several other categories, will receive punishment in a *"fiery lake of burning sulfur"* (Revelation 21:8). Whether viewed literally or metaphorically, that's a bad scene.

Hanging beside the toilet in the bathroom of my childhood home was a razor strap. In those days my Dad was moving away from the old straight edge razor to the revolutionary new Gillette "blue blades." The razor strap had a continuing function, however. Its purpose was to be a deterrent to disobedience. Funny thing, it worked. None of us was perfect and so we all got some swats from the razor strap, but to go in there and see the leather strap hanging benignly on the wall reminded me that I wanted it to stay there. Proverbs declared the *"fear of the LORD is the beginning of wisdom"* (1:7). It is wise to know that God is serious about His "line drawn in the sand." There is an awful price to pay for defiance of God.

One might ask at this point, where is the church in all of this. It seems that in all divisions of the Christian church immorality surfaces among those who are expected to demonstrate a life that honors Jesus and righteousness. Something is askew in the church itself. Historically, church leadership has not understood the significance or the spiritual power available to live godly sexual lives.

The spirit is humanity's link with God, his creator and Savior. The spirit is the source of meaning and purpose. It directs values and priorities and behavior. Love is first spiritual, the meaningful commitment of two people to one another in a permanent relationship. It is the ultimate expression of acceptance and trust. Sex is to flow out of that spiritual fountain.

12

THE ROLE OF THE CHURCH

If there is any place in the whole world where we ought to be honest, it is in the church of God.[90]

Husbands, love your wives, just as Christ loved the church and gave himself up for her to make her holy, cleansing her by the washing with water through the word, and to present her to himself as a radiant church, without stain or wrinkle or any other blemish, but holy and blameless (Ephesians 5:25-27 NIV).

Husbands, go all out in your love for your wives, exactly as Christ did for the church—a love marked by giving, not getting. Christ's love makes the church whole. His words evoke her beauty. Everything he does and says is designed to bring the best out of her, dressing her in dazzling white silk, radiant with holiness (The Message).

That sex has brought consternation to the church is not confined to the Victorian period or to continued awkwardness in the twenty-first century. Peter Brown researched the church's attempts to address the subject in his exhaustive study in *The*

---

90   Harry Verploegh, *The Quotable Tozer* (Original published as *A. W. Tozer: An Anthology*), 1994, Quick Verse.

Body and Society: Men, Women, and Sexual Renunciation in Early Christianity. One view was that of Stoicism. "For the Stoics, intercourse was supposed to take place only so as to produce children. *The couple must not make love for the sake of pleasure alone; even the positions that they adopted should only be those that enabled the seed to be 'sown' to best effect.*"[91] *Christians did not escape the cultural understanding. "Certain restraints that came to be advocated in Christian circles rested lightly on upper-class males. The well-too-do Greek or Roman was a slave-owner. Men owned the bodies of their male and female servants. Within the walls of a great rambling house, filled with young servants, over whom the master ruled supreme, fidelity to one's wife remained a personal option."*[92] *The early church, Brown demonstrated, put a premium on sexual restraint, but the emphasis was not on spiritual transformation; it was on rules and laws to restrain behavior.*

The Use of Dogma to Instigate and to Control Behavior

Most people lose or forget the subjectively religious experience, and redefine Religion as a set of habits, behaviors, dogmas, forms, which at the extreme becomes entirely legalistic and bureaucratic, conventional, empty, and in the truest meaning of the word, anti-religious. The mystic experience, the illuminations, the great awakening, along with the charismatic seer who started the whole thing, are forgotten, lost, or transformed into their opposites. Organized religion, the churches, finally may become the major enemies of the religious experience and the religious experiencer.[93]

---

91   Brown, 21.

92   *Ibid.*, 23.

93   Abraham Hl Maslow, *Religion, Values, and Peak-Experiences* (New York: The Viking Press, 1964), viii.

The most immediate response to the decline of spiritual vitality
is to formulate a law or rule that prohibits a specific practice. That
is based on the assumption that the source of the error is the error
itself. Both the Scriptures and history repudiate such a claim.
Hebrews declares that a sinful heart is one that "turns away from the
living God" (3:12). That willful act produces a tragic spiritual decline
that eventuates in various sinful behaviors. Although this is
biblically evident, the church ignored it and turned to making rules.

Ezra was acutely aware of the spiritual inconsistencies of his
people in previous centuries. Their apathy and sinfulness had brought
God's judgment destroying first the northern kingdom and later the
southern kingdom. Ezra was the first to return from Babylonian
captivity and was later followed by Nehemiah. He was a scribe who
knew the law and was the instigator of massive reforms among the
people by confronting the people with the law of God. The reforms
affected not only the worship practices but even resulted in the
dissolving of mixed marriages, illegal in the Jewish culture.

John Bright concluded that "it is not incorrect to regard him
[Ezra] as the father of Judaism."[94] With Ezra, the prophetic
movement became subject to the emphasis upon law. "The law,
indeed, took over the function of prophecy: that of stating the
Word of God."[95] Had the lawyers limited themselves to God's law,
they would have retained prophetic life. Rather, it became the
very essence of religion "to study the law, discuss it, teach it, keep
it. And since every law needs definition…there was need for further
rulings to give the needed clarification."[96] In time the definitions

---

94   John Bright, *The Kingdom of God* (Nashville: Abingdon Press, 1953),
174.
95   *Ibid.*
96   *Ibid.*, 175.

became equal to God's laws and hundreds of legislations made an intolerable burden.

There was Nothing Malicious in the Desired Goal.

"The law sought to create the true people of God over whom God could establish his rule. The end of the law was never rule keeping for the rule's sake; it was God, and total obedience to God."[97] What was not the desired end (rule keeping) became in fact the end. Rule is inevitable when men bypass the basis of spiritual renewal through a divine encounter and establish rules of their own making those rules equal to God's Word. Rule keeping is nothing less than human merit to gain credibility with God. All such attempts are futile and the letters of Paul express the adamant wrath of God against such.

In contrast to rule keeping, righteousness is "total dedication to the will of the Father.... Righteousness is therefore no longer an external conformity, but an inwardly motivated obedience which 'fulfills' the law."[98]

The history of the church is a cycle of repeated attempts to control behavior through rules, intimidation, anathema and other degenerate forms of manipulative discipline. Unless evangelism is kept central in its declaration of transforming as well as saving power, the abuses of institutionalism are inevitable.

For two millenniums the church has been convening in councils to discuss matters of faith and of disciplinary decrees. In a massive work on the disciplinary decrees of these general councils H. J. Schroeder confirmed that "most of the councils held by the

---

97   *Ibid.*, 176.
98   *Ibid.*, 205.

Church in the course of her history, whether ecumenical or provincial, formed it a matter of necessity to issue series of disciplinary measures or rules, designed for the good of government of Christian society and the sanctification of individuals."[99]

The stance of the Roman church is that "the resultant decisions or decrees of these councils are invested with the authority of the entire assembly, are after papal confirmation binding on all the faithful."[100]

A doctrinal problem that had divided the church was a basic concern in the Council of Nicaea held in 325 A.D. The teaching called the Arian heresy denied the divinity of Christ. That this is a basic issue, no orthodox Christian would deny. The heretics based their argument on the ground that there is only one God and that he cannot have a Son equal to Himself being of the same substance for that would imply divisibility. The Word, they argued, is a creature, the first and the most perfect that was neither God nor a part of the world. Through His sinless life He merited adoption by God as His Son and so is thereby worthy of worship.

In repudiation of this devastating Christology, the creed declared:

> *Those who say: there was a time when He was not, and He was not before He was begotten, and that He was made out of nothing; or who say that He is of another hypostasis or another substance (than the Father), or that the Son of God is created or is susceptible of change or alteration, (them) the Catholic and Apostolic Church anathematizes.*[101]

---

99   Rev. H. J. Schroeder, o.p., *Disciplinary Decrees of the General Councils* (St. Louis, MO: B. Herder Book Co., 1937), 1.

100   5.

101   16.

Such a creedal decree is well within the claims and statements of New Testament doctrine. It neither intimidates nor manipulates but simply emphasizes biblical doctrine.

The council did not stop with that consideration. It also established twenty canons of discipline. Voluntary eunuchs were excluded from the ministry unless their surgery was for medical purposes. New converts were not allowed to be promoted to sacerdotal or episcopal positions. No one in any order of ministry was to have a woman other than a close relative living with him. "The purpose of the canon was to put an end to a moral disorder that had developed among the clergy."[102] Jurisdictional issues were resolved. Priests who were guilty of certain sins before their ordination were to be disposed. The sins included adultery, homicide, blasphemy, bigamy, heresy, etc.

People who had apostatized during the severe persecution of Licinius were required to do twelve years of penance but those who were dying while under discipline were allowed to be given Eucharist. Clergymen were not allowed to charge interest for loans. A precise order and sequence for serving Eucharist was established prohibiting deacons from serving priests. And, as though important, from Easter to Pentecost, prayers could be said *standing!*[103]

The ensuing councils record additional and repeated canons. Several councils had to restate the ejection of priests guilty of immorality,[104] the banning of priest's sons from the priesthood,[105] (evidently the law wasn't too effective), and nuns were prevented

---

102   *Ibid.*, 22.
103   8-58.
104   496.
105   208.

from marrying.[106] The rules failed to curb immoral sex. Also such weighty matters as the anathematizing of slingers and archers who warred against Christians was decreed along with charging priests to refrain from getting drunk.[107] Anyone who punched a priest in the nose (*i.e.* laid violent hands on him) was subject to being anathematized.[108] Some clerics were not allowed "to cultivate long hair or a beard; neither shall they have horses and mules with coverings and ornaments made of velvet or silk."[109] Century after century, council after council rules were written to control behavior or establish discipline for previously broken rules. They did not change hearts.

Man is a sinful creature, and behavioral controls without behavioral change through regeneration and the filling of the Spirit can only be manipulative. This applies not only to matters of sexual ethics but of all areas of morality and spiritual vitality.

Now, nearly two millenniums later, we are still subject to the influence of cultural norms that view sex as something that is highly personal and subject to the individual's determination of right or wrong. The general norm is that living together before marriage is comparable to test driving a car before buying. Dr. Phil summarized diverse data on marriage and divorce.

106	213.
107	256.
108	204.
109	495.

Marriage and Divorce: The Statistics

Learn what the 2003 data reveals about who is getting married, when they're getting married, and who is most likely to divorce.

- The average age of a woman getting married in the United States is 27. *" Bride's Magazine*

- The average age of a man getting married in the United States is 29. *" Bride's Magazine*

- 88 percent of American men and women between the ages of 20 and 29 believe that they have a soul mate who is waiting for them. *" University Wire, Louisiana State University*

- 59 percent of marriages for women under the age of 18 end in divorce within 15 years. The divorce rate drops to 36 percent for those married at age 20 or older. *" "Cohabitation, Marriage, Divorce and Remarriage in the United States," M.D. Bramlett and W.D. Mosher*

- 60 percent of marriages for couples between the ages of 20 and 25 end in divorce. *" National Center for Health Statistics*

- 50 percent of all marriages in which the brides are 25 or older result in a failed marriage. *" National Center for Health Statistics*

- 65 percent of altar-bound men and women live together before getting married. *" Bride's Magazine*

- Research indicates that people who live together prior to getting married are more likely to have marriages that end in divorce. *" The Boston Herald*

- A recent study on cohabitation concluded that after five to seven years, only 21 percent of unmarried couples were still living together. *" The Boston Herald*

- 55 percent of cohabitating couples get married within five years of moving in together. Forty percent of couples who live together break up within that same time period. *" Annual Review of Sociology*

- Children of divorce have a higher risk of divorce when they marry and an even higher risk if the person they marry comes from a divorced home. One study found that when the wife alone had experienced a parental divorce, her odds of divorce increased to 59 percent. When both spouses experienced parental divorce, the odds of divorce nearly tripled to 189 percent. *" Journal of Marriage and the Family*

- The likelihood that a woman will eventually marry is significantly lower for those who first had a child out of wedlock. By age 35, only 70 percent of all unwed mothers are married in contrast to 88 percent of women who have not had a child out of wedlock. " *"Finding a Mate? The Marital and Cohabitation Histories of Unwed Mothers," Lawrence L. Wu and Barbara Wolfe*[110]

Sex is the most widely practiced activity and least talked about subject in the church. Evangelical Christians complain about sex education in the public system, state it belongs in the home and then systematically avoid addressing the subject. Little is offered to assist parents in discussing the subject with their children and much too little is given to teach children and students a biblical perspective on the subject. Branches within the Christian church have opted to redefine Scripture and approve the ordination of homosexual clergy and conducting same sex marriages. What the church could have explained as a parable of God's love and character has been left open

---

110   http://www.drphil.com/articles/article/351, (accessed August 15, 2013).

as a playground of the devil. The biblical relationship of a husband and wife fosters the best environment for healthy sex. The church has simply echoed the "just say no" slogan, which clearly hasn't worked. Church education must teach biblical, healthy sex.

Paul did not hesitate to address this issue. The church in Corinth had a real sticky problem. A member of the church was having an affair with his step-mother. Nothing was done to correct the situation. The church actually took pride in its liberal stance of acceptance. In the same direct and strong terms of the ancient Hebrew law, Paul confronted the church and demanded them to:

> …hand this man over to Satan, so that the sinful nature may be destroyed and his spirit saved on the day of the Lord. Your boasting is not good. Don't you know that a little yeast works through the whole batch of dough? Get rid of the old yeast that you may be a new batch without yeast—as you really are…. I have written you in my letter not to associate with sexually immoral people—not at all meaning the people of this world who are immoral, or the greedy and swindlers, or idolaters. In that case you would have to leave this world. But now I am writing you that you must not associate with anyone who calls himself a brother but is sexually immoral… (1 Corinthians 5:5-7, 9-11).

That seems like very harsh medicine in a culture where tolerance is the supreme virtue. However, tolerance is not synonymous with love. It is more self-love than concern for others. Tolerance only has value in view of what is not tolerated. Not all forms of belief or behavior are of equal value. The law of society rejects some behaviors and accepts others. If every act were equally acceptable, our streets and homes would be much less safe than now.

Can Church Dogma Change or Control Behavior?

> Since you died with Christ to the basic principles of this world, why, as though you still belonged to it, do you submit to its rules: "Do not handle! Do not taste! Do not touch!"? These are all destined to perish with use, because they are based on human commands and teachings. Such regulations indeed have an appearance of wisdom, with their self-imposed worship, their false humility and their harsh treatment of the body, but they lack any value in restraining sensual indulgence (Colossians 2:20-23 NIV).

Attempts to control the lusts of the heart through religious ritual will only result in frustration and defeat. Change must come from the inside from the personal presence of the Holy Spirit who alone provides the inner power of restraint to avoid sin. Psychology might identify some of the emotional longings a person seeks in sexual involvement but it is powerless to come inside the person and change or bring healing. Philosophical concepts can express noble intent and inspire a positive response; in finality they are human thoughts. The Holy Spirit is the master of behavioral change. Paul prayed that the Father

> ...may strengthen you with power through his Spirit in your inner being, so that Christ may dwell in your hearts through faith. And I pray that you being rooted and established in love, may have power...to grasp how wide and long and high and deep is the love of Christ, and to know this love that surpasses knowledge—that you may be filled to the measure of all the fullness of God (Ephesians 3:16-19 NIV).

Good News—the Gospel

God is the source of grace and healing. The psalmist celebrated: "He heals the brokenhearted and binds up their wounds" (Psalm 147:3). Isaiah in writing the gospel of the Old Testament stated, "Although the Lord gives you the bread of adversity and the water of affliction, your teachers will be hidden no more; with your own eyes you will see them. Whether you turn to right or to the left, your ears will hear a voice behind you, saying, 'This is the way; walk in it....' The moon will shine like the sun, and the sunlight will be seven times brighter, like the light of seven full days, when the LORD binds up the bruises of his people and heals the wounds he inflicted" (30:20-21, 26). Forecasting the coming of Jesus as Messiah, Isaiah assures us, "A bruised reed he will not break, and a smoldering wick he will not snuff out" (42:3).

Everyone is guilty of sexual sin, either in mental lust or taking the mental to physical behavior. Jesus said if a man looks with lust on a woman, he is guilty of adultery. He also said of the woman caught by religious phonies in the act of adultery and so wanted her stoned, let the one without sin throw the first stone. They all silently slithered away. Forgiveness is yours. Take it. The Holy Spirit is available; give Him control and learn to walk in step with Him.

Prayer for Purity

O Thou, to whose all-searching sight
The darkness shineth as the light,
Search, prove my heart; it pants for Thee;
O burst these bonds, and set it free!

Wash out its stains, refine its dross,
Nail my affections to the Cross;
Hallow each thought; let all within
Be clean, as Thou, my Lord, art clean!

If in this darksome wild I stray,
Be Thou my Light, be Thou my Way;
No foes, no violence I fear,
No fraud, while Thou, my God, art near.

When rising floods my soul o'erflow,
When sinks my heart in waves of woe,
Jesus, Thy timely aid impart,
And raise my head, and cheer my heart.

Saviour, where'er Thy steps I see,
Dauntless, untired, I follow Thee;
O let Thy hand support me still,
And lead me to Thy holy hill!

If rough and thorny be the way,
My strength proportion to my day;
Till toil, and grief, and pain shall cease,
Where all is calm, and joy, and peace.

Nicolaus Ludwig von Zinzendort (1700-1760)
Tr. John Wesley, (1703-1791)[111]

---

111   A. W. Tozer, *The Christian Book of Mystical Verse* (Harrisburg, PA: Christian Publications, Inc., 1963), 46-47.

"I am certain that God,
who began the good work within you
will continue his work until it is finally finished
on the day when Christ Jesus returns."

(Philippians 1:6 NLT).

ABOUT THE AUTHOR

Roy C. Price, DMin, DPhil, is a graduate of Westmont College in English Literature, Luther Rice Seminary (ThM, DMin), and Oxford Graduate School, USA. (DPhil in the sociological integration of religion and society.) He presently serves as Adjunct Professor of Pastoral Theology and Polity at the A. W. Tozer Theological Seminary, Redding, CA.

Dr. Price served various pastorates with a missionary attitude. His ministry included experience in rural, suburban, urban, and international congregations. He served in several regional elected positions of his denomination and two terms on the Board of Directors of the national organization of the Christian and Missionary Alliance. Dr. Price also served on the Board of Regents of Oxford Graduate School, USA. Significant articles have appeared in Leadership magazine, Christianity Today, and the Alliance Life magazine. Roy and his wife live in northern California near their grandchildren.

God and the Sexual Metaphor, is a timely book that brings a Judeo-Christian biblical world view to the issues of human sexuality. The assumption is that God designed sex, not man or society, and that human sexual expression in the context of marriage is good in the sight of God. Dr. Price believes the Bible is a guide to human behavior which includes sexual expression. He also affirms that there are benefits in conforming to God's guidelines and consequences when one does not conform. He believes human beings are born in a sinful condition that can be changed by a relationship with Jesus Christ. Pastors, parents, youth and youth workers will benefit from the study of *God and the Sexual Metaphor*, which is the sharing of a spiritual father's understanding.

Selected Bibliography

Barclay, William. *A New Testament* Wordbook. New York: Harper & Brothers. n.d.

———. *The Letters of James and Peter*. Philadelphia: The Westminster Press, 1958.

———. *More New Testament Words*. New York: Harper & Brothers Publishers, 1958.

Baxter, J. Sidlow. *A New Call to Holiness*. Grand Rapids, MI: Zondervan Publishing House, 1973.

Bright, John. *The Kingdom of God: the Biblical concept and its meaning for the church*. Nashville: Abingdon Press, 1953.

Brown, Colin, General Editor. *The New International Dictionary of New Testament Theology*. Grand Rapids, Michigan: Zondervan Publishing House, 1978.

Brown, Peter. *The Body and Society: Men, Women, and Sexual Renunciation in Early Christianity*. New York: Columbia University Press.

Buchanan, Mark. *Hidden in Plain Sight: the Secret of More*. Nashville, TN: Thomas Nelson, Inc., 2007.

Drummond, Henry. *The Greatest Thing in the World*. Westwood, New Jersey: Fleming H. Revell Company, n. d.

Feinberg, John S and Paul D. Feinberg. *Ethics for a Brave New World*. Wheaton, Illinois: Crossway Books, 1993

Freligh, Harold M. *The Eight Pillars of Salvation*. Minneapolis, Minnesota: Bethany Fellowship, Inc., 1962.

Grenz, Stanley J. David Guretzki, Cherith Fee Nordling. *Pocket Dictionary of Theological Terms*. Copyright © 1999. All rights reserved, Electronic Edition STEP Files Copyright © 2007, QuickVerse.

Harrris, R. Laird, ed., *Theological Wordbook of the Old Testament*. Chicago: Moody Press, 1980.

Henry, Carl F. H. *Christian Personal Ethics*. Grand Rapids, MI: Wm B. Eerdmans Publishing Co, 1957.

Johnson, Paul. *The Intellectuals*. New York: Harper & Row, Publishers, 1988.

Jones, S. L. "Sexuality," Benner, David G, Peter C Hill. *Baker Encyclopedia of Psychology*. Grand Rapids, Mich.: Baker Books, 1985.

Keely, Robin ed. *Eerdmans' Handbook to Christian Belief*. Grand Rapids, Michigan: Wm B. Eerdmans Publishing Co., 1982.

Kittel, Gerhard, and Gerhard Friedrich ed., translated by Geoffrey W. Bromiley. Abridged by Geoffrey W. Bromiley. *Theological Dictionary of the New Testament*. Grand Rapids, Mich.: William B. Eerdmans Publishing Company. 1985. Electronic Edition STEP Files Copyright © 2007, Findex.Com.

Maslow, Abraham H. *Religion, Values, and Peak-Experiences*. New York: The Viking Press, 1964.

McGrath, Alister E. *Christian Theology: An Introduction*. University of Oxford: Blackwell Publishing, 2007.

Orr, James, M.A., D.D., General Editor Parsons Technology, Inc. Cedar Rapids, Iowa *International Standard Bible Encyclopedia*, "Know, Knowledge," "Agape" Electronic Edition STEP Files Copyright © 1998, Parsons Technology, Inc.

Packer, James. *Your Father Loves You: Daily Insights for Knowing God*. Compiled and edited by Jean Watson. Wheaton, Illinois: Harold Shaw Publishers, 1986.

Paterson, James and Peter Kim. *The Day America Told the Truth*. New York: Prentice Hall Press, 1991.

Payne, J. Barton. *The Theology of the Older Testament*. Grand Rapids, Michigan: Zondervan Publishing House, 1962.

Rienecker, Fritz and Cleon Rogers. *Linguistic Key to the Greek New Testament*. Grand Rapids, MI: Regency Reference Library, 1980.

Schroeder, Rev. H. J. o.p. *Disciplinary Decrees of the General Councils*. St. Louis, MO: B. Herder Book Co., 1937.

Smedes, Lewis B. "The Changing Sexual Scene," Robin Keeley, ed., *Christianity in Today's World* (Grand Rapids, Michigan: Wm B. Eerdmans Publishing Co., 1985

Thiessen, Henry Clarence. *Introductory Lectures in Systematic Theology.* Grand Rapids, Michigan: Wm. B. Eerdmans Publishing Co, 1975.

Tozer, A. W. *The Christian Book of Mystical Verse.* Harrisburg, PA: Christian Publications, Inc., 1963.

——. *Man the Dwelling Place of God.* Camp Hill, PA: Christian Publications, 1966.

——. Tozer, *The Attributes of God: A Journey into the Father's Heart.* Camp Hill, PA, Christian Publications, Inc., 1997. QuickVerse e-publication.

Young, Sarah. *Jesus Calling: Enjoying Peace in His Presence.* Nashville, Tennessee: Thomas Nelson, 2004.

Verploegh, Harry. *The Quotable Tozer.* Original published as *A. W. Tozer: An Anthology,* 1994. QuickVerse.

APPENDIX

Appearance of prostitute, adultery and related words

Genesis 34:31 (NIV)
But they replied, "Should he have treated our sister like a prostitute?"

Genesis 38:15 (NIV)
When Judah saw her, he thought she was a prostitute, for she had covered her face.

Genesis 38:21 (NIV)
He asked the men who lived there, "Where is the shrine prostitute who was beside the road at Enaim?" "There hasn't been any shrine prostitute here," they said.

Genesis 38:22 (NIV)
So he went back to Judah and said, "I didn't find her. Besides, the men who lived there said, 'There hasn't been any shrine prostitute here.'"

Genesis 38:24 (NIV)
About three months later Judah was told, "Your daughter-in-law Tamar is guilty of prostitution, and as a result she is now pregnant." Judah said, "Bring her out and have her burned to death!"

Exodus 20:14 (NIV)
You shall not commit adultery.

Exodus 34:15 (NIV)
"Be careful not to make a treaty with those who live in the land; for when they prostitute themselves to their gods and sacrifice to them, they will invite you and you will eat their sacrifices.

Exodus 34:16 (NIV)
And when you choose some of their daughters as wives for your sons and those daughters prostitute themselves to their gods, they will lead your sons to do the same.

Leviticus 17:7 (NIV)
They must no longer offer any of their sacrifices to the goat idols to whom they prostitute themselves. This is to be a lasting ordinance for them and for the generations to come.'

Leviticus 19:29 (NIV)
Do not degrade your daughter by making her a prostitute, or the land will turn to prostitution and be filled with wickedness.

Leviticus 20:5 (NIV)
I will set my face against that man and his family and will cut off from their people both him and all who follow him in prostituting themselves to Molech.

Leviticus 20:6 (NIV)
'I will set my face against the person who turns to mediums and spiritists to prostitute himself by following them, and I will cut him off from his people.

Leviticus 20:10 (NIV)
If a man commits adultery with another man's wife--with the wife of his neighbor--both the adulterer and the adulteress must be put to death.

Leviticus 20:10 (NIV)
If a man commits adultery with another man's wife--with the wife of his neighbor--both the adulterer and the adulteress must be put to death.

Leviticus 20:10 (NIV)
If a man commits adultery with another man's wife--with the wife of his neighbor--both the adulterer and the adulteress must be put to death.

Leviticus 21:7 (NIV)
They must not marry women defiled by prostitution or divorced from their husbands, because priests are holy to their God.

Leviticus 21:9 (NIV)
If a priest's daughter defiles herself by becoming a prostitute, she disgraces her father; she must be burned in the fire.

Leviticus 21:14 (NIV)
He must not marry a widow, a divorced woman, or a woman defiled by prostitution, but only a virgin from his own people,

Numbers 15:39 (NIV)
You will have these tassels to look at and so you will remember all the

commands of the LORD, that you may obey them and not prostitute yourselves by going after the lusts of your own hearts and eyes.

Deuteronomy 5:18 (NIV)
You shall not commit adultery.

Deuteronomy 23:17 (NIV)
No Israelite man or woman is to become a shrine prostitute.

Deuteronomy 23:18 (NIV)
You must not bring the earnings of a female prostitute or of a male prostitute into the house of the LORD your God to pay any vow, because the LORD your God detests them both.

Deuteronomy 31:16 (NIV)
And the LORD said to Moses: "You are going to rest with your fathers, and these people will soon prostitute themselves to the foreign gods of the land they are entering. They will forsake me and break the covenant I made with them.

Joshua 2:1 (NIV)
Then Joshua son of Nun secretly sent two spies from Shittim. "Go, look over the land," he said, "especially Jericho." So they went and entered the house of a prostitute named Rahab and stayed there.

Joshua 6:17 (NIV)
The city and all that is in it are to be devoted to the LORD. Only Rahab the prostitute and all who are with her in her house shall be spared, because she hid the spies we sent.

Joshua 6:25 (NIV)
But Joshua spared Rahab the prostitute, with her family and all who belonged to her, because she hid the men Joshua had sent as spies to Jericho--and she lives among the Israelites to this day.

Judges 2:17 (NIV)
Yet they would not listen to their judges but prostituted themselves to other gods and worshiped them. Unlike their fathers, they quickly turned from the way in which their fathers had walked, the way of obedience to the LORD's commands.

Judges 8:27 (NIV)
Gideon made the gold into an ephod, which he placed in Ophrah, his town. All Israel prostituted themselves by worshiping it there, and it became a snare to Gideon and his family.

Judges 8:33 (NIV)
No sooner had Gideon died than the Israelites again prostituted themselves to the Baals. They set up Baal-Berith as their god and

Judges 11:1 (NIV)
Jephthah the Gileadite was a mighty warrior. His father was Gilead; his mother was a prostitute.

Judges 16:1 (NIV)
One day Samson went to Gaza, where he saw a prostitute. He went in to spend the night with her.

1 Kings 3:16 (NIV)
Now two prostitutes came to the king and stood before him.

1 Kings 14:24 (NIV)
There were even male shrine prostitutes in the land; the people engaged in all the detestable practices of the nations the LORD had driven out before the Israelites.

1 Kings 15:12 (NIV)
He expelled the male shrine prostitutes from the land and got rid of all the idols his fathers had made.

1 Kings 22:38 (NIV)
They washed the chariot at a pool in Samaria (where the prostitutes bathed), and the dogs licked up his blood, as the word of the LORD had declared.

1 Kings 22:46 (NIV)
He rid the land of the rest of the male shrine prostitutes who remained there even after the reign of his father Asa.

2 Kings 23:7 (NIV)
He also tore down the quarters of the male shrine prostitutes, which were in the temple of the LORD and where women did weaving for Asherah.

1 Chronicles 5:25 (NIV)
But they were unfaithful to the God of their fathers and prostituted themselves to the gods of the peoples of the land, whom God had destroyed before them.

2 Chronicles 21:11 (NIV)
He had also built high places on the hills of Judah and had caused the people of Jerusalem to prostitute themselves and had led Judah astray.

2 Chronicles 21:13 (NIV)
But you have walked in the ways of the kings of Israel, and you have led Judah and the people of Jerusalem to prostitute themselves, just as the house of Ahab did. You have also murdered your own brothers, members of your father's house, men who were better than you.

Job 36:14 (NIV)
They die in their youth, among male prostitutes of the shrines.

Psalm 50:18 (NIV)
When you see a thief, you join with him; you throw in your lot with adulterers.

Psalm 66:5 (NIV)
Come and see what God has done, how awesome his works in man's behalf!

Psalm 76:8 (NIV)
From heaven you pronounced judgment, and the land feared and was quiet--

Psalm 77:1 (NIV)
I cried out to God for help; I cried out to God to hear me.

Psalm 77:2 (NIV)
When I was in distress, I sought the Lord; at night I stretched out untiring hands and my soul refused to be comforted.

Psalm 77:16 (NIV)
The waters saw you, O God, the waters saw you and writhed; the very depths were convulsed.

Psalm 106:39 (NIV)
They defiled themselves by what they did; by their deeds they prostituted themselves.

Proverbs 2:16 (NIV)
It will save you also from the adulteress, from the wayward wife with her seductive words,

Proverbs 5:3 (NIV)
For the lips of an adulteress drip honey, and her speech is smoother than oil;

Proverbs 5:20 (NIV)
Why be captivated, my son, by an adulteress? Why embrace the bosom of another man's wife?

Proverbs 6:26 (NIV)
for the prostitute reduces you to a loaf of bread, and the adulteress preys upon your very life.

Proverbs 6:32 (NIV)
But a man who commits adultery lacks judgment; whoever does so destroys himself.

Proverbs 7:5 (NIV)
They will keep you from the adulteress, from the wayward wife with her seductive words.

Proverbs 7:10 (NIV)
Then out came a woman to meet him, dressed like a prostitute and with crafty intent.

Proverbs 22:14 (NIV)
The mouth of an adulteress is a deep pit; he who is under the LORD's wrath will fall into it.

Proverbs 23:27 (NIV)
For a prostitute is a deep pit and a wayward wife is a narrow well.

Proverbs 29:3 (NIV)
A man who loves wisdom brings joy to his father, but a companion of prostitutes squanders his wealth.

Proverbs 30:20 (NIV)
This is the way of an adulteress: She eats and wipes her mouth and says, 'I've done nothing wrong.'

Isaiah 23:15 (NIV)
At that time Tyre will be forgotten for seventy years, the span of a king's life. But at the end of these seventy years, it will happen to Tyre as in the song of the prostitute:

Isaiah 23:16 (NIV)
"Take up a harp, walk through the city, O prostitute forgotten; play the harp well, sing many a song, so that you will be remembered."

Isaiah 23:17 (NIV)
At the end of seventy years, the LORD will deal with Tyre. She will return to her hire as a prostitute and will ply her trade with all the kingdoms on the face of the earth.

Isaiah 57:3 (NIV)
But you--come here, you sons of a sorceress, you offspring of adulterers and prostitutes!

Jeremiah 2:20 (NIV)
Long ago you broke off your yoke and tore off your bonds; you said, 'I will not serve you!' Indeed, on every high hill and under every spreading tree you lay down as a prostitute.

Jeremiah 3:1 (NIV)
"If a man divorces his wife and she leaves him and marries another man, should he return to her again? Would not the land be completely defiled? But you have lived as a prostitute with many lovers-- would you now return to me?" declares the LORD.

Jeremiah 3:2 (NIV)
Look up to the barren heights and see. Is there any place where you have not been ravished? By the roadside you sat waiting for lovers, sat like a nomad in the desert. You have defiled the land with your prostitution and wickedness.

Jeremiah 3:3 (NIV)
Therefore the showers have been withheld, and no spring rains have fallen. Yet you have the brazen look of a prostitute; you refuse to blush with shame.

Jeremiah 3:6 (NIV)
During the reign of King Josiah, the LORD said to me, "Have you seen what faithless Israel has done? She has gone up on every high hill and under every spreading tree and has committed adultery there."

Jeremiah 3:8 (NIV)
I gave faithless Israel her certificate of divorce and sent her away because of all her adulteries. Yet I saw that her unfaithful sister Judah had no fear; she also went out and committed adultery.

Jeremiah 3:8 (NIV)
I gave faithless Israel her certificate of divorce and sent her away because of all her adulteries. Yet I saw that her unfaithful sister Judah had no fear; she also went out and committed adultery.

Jeremiah 3:9 (NIV)
Because Israel's immorality mattered so little to her, she defiled the land and committed adultery with stone and wood.

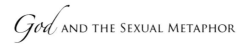

Jeremiah 5:7 (NIV)
Why should I forgive you? Your children have forsaken me and sworn by gods that are not gods. I supplied all their needs, yet they committed adultery and thronged to the houses of prostitutes.

Jeremiah 7:9 (NIV)
Will you steal and murder, commit adultery and perjury, burn incense to Baal and follow other gods you have not known,

Jeremiah 13:27 (NIV)
Your adulteries and lustful neighings, your shameless prostitution! I have seen your detestable acts on the hills and in the fields. Woe to you, O Jerusalem! How long will you be unclean?"

Jeremiah 23:14 (NIV)
And among the prophets of Jerusalem I have seen something horrible: They commit adultery and live a lie. They strengthen the hands of evildoers, so that no one turns from his wickedness. They are all like Sodom to me; the people of Jerusalem are like Gomorrah.

Jeremiah 29:23 (NIV)
For they have done outrageous things in Israel; they have committed adultery with their neighbors' wives and in my name have spoken lies, which I did not tell them to do. I know it and am a witness to it," declares the LORD.

Ezekiel 6:9 (NIV)
Then in the nations where they have been carried captive, those who escape will remember me--how I have been grieved by their adulterous hearts, which have turned away from me, and by their eyes, which have lusted after their idols. They will loathe themselves for the evil they have done and for all their detestable practices.

Ezekiel 16:15-17 (NIV)
But you trusted in your beauty and used your fame to become a prostitute. You lavished your favors on anyone who passed by and your beauty became his. You took some of your garments to make gaudy high places, where you carried on your prostitution. Such things should not happen, nor should they ever occur. You also took the fine jewelry I gave you, the jewelry made of my gold and silver, and you made for yourself male idols and engaged in prostitution with them.

Ezekiel 16:20 (NIV)
And you took your sons and daughters whom you bore to me and sacrificed them as food to the idols. Was your prostitution not enough?

Ezekiel 16:22 (NIV)
In all your detestable practices and your prostitution you did not remember
the days of your youth, when you were naked and bare, kicking about in
your blood.

Ezekiel 16:26 (NIV)
You engaged in prostitution with the Egyptians, your lustful neighbors, and
provoked me to anger with your increasing promiscuity.

Ezekiel 16:28 (NIV)
You engaged in prostitution with the Assyrians too, because you were
insatiable; and even after that, you still were not satisfied.

Ezekiel 16:30-35 (NIV)
How weak-willed you are, declares the Sovereign LORD, when you do all
these things, acting like a brazen prostitute! When you built your mounds at
the head of every street and made your lofty shrines in every public square,
you were unlike a prostitute, because you scorned payment. You adulterous
wife! You prefer strangers to your own husband! Every prostitute receives
a fee, but you give gifts to all your lovers, bribing them to come to you
from everywhere for your illicit favors. So in your prostitution you are the
opposite of others; no one runs after you for your favors. You are the very
opposite, for you give payment and none is given to you. Therefore, you
prostitute, hear the word of the LORD!

Ezekiel 16:38 (NIV)
I will sentence you to the punishment of women who commit adultery and
who shed blood; I will bring upon you the blood vengeance of my wrath
and jealous anger.

Ezekiel 16:41 (NIV)
They will burn down your houses and inflict punishment on you in the
sight of many women. I will put a stop to your prostitution, and you will no
longer pay your lovers.

Ezekiel 23:3 (NIV)
They became prostitutes in Egypt, engaging in prostitution from their youth.
In that land their breasts were fondled and their virgin bosoms caressed.

Ezekiel 23:5 (NIV)
Oholah engaged in prostitution while she was still mine; and she lusted after
her lovers, the Assyrians--warriors

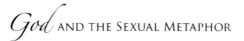

Ezekiel 23:7 (NIV)
She gave herself as a prostitute to all the elite of the Assyrians and defiled herself with all the idols of everyone she lusted after.

Ezekiel 23:8 (NIV)
She did not give up the prostitution she began in Egypt, when during her youth men slept with her, caressed her virgin bosom and poured out their lust upon her.

Ezekiel 23:11 (NIV)
Her sister Oholibah saw this, yet in her lust and prostitution she was more depraved than her sister.

Ezekiel 23:14 (NIV)
But she carried her prostitution still further. She saw men portrayed on a wall, figures of Chaldeans portrayed in red,

Ezekiel 23:18-19 (NIV)
When she carried on her prostitution openly and exposed her nakedness, I turned away from her in disgust, just as I had turned away from her sister. Yet she became more and more promiscuous as she recalled the days of her youth, when she was a prostitute in Egypt.

Ezekiel 23:27 (NIV)
So I will put a stop to the lewdness and prostitution you began in Egypt. You will not look on these things with longing or remember Egypt anymore.

Ezekiel 23:29 (NIV)
They will deal with you in hatred and take away everything you have worked for. They will leave you naked and bare, and the shame of your prostitution will be exposed. Your lewdness and promiscuity

Ezekiel 23:35 (NIV)
Therefore this is what the Sovereign LORD says: Since you have forgotten me and thrust me behind your back, you must bear the consequences of your lewdness and prostitution."

Ezekiel 23:37 (NIV)
For they have committed adultery and blood is on their hands. They committed adultery with their idols; they even sacrificed their children, whom they bore to me, as food for them.

Ezekiel 23:43 (NIV)
Then I said about the one worn out by adultery, 'Now let them use her as a prostitute, for that is all she is.'

Ezekiel 23:44 (NIV)
And they slept with her. As men sleep with a prostitute, so they slept with those lewd women, Oholah and Oholibah.

Ezekiel 23:45 (NIV)
But righteous men will sentence them to the punishment of women who commit adultery and shed blood, because they are adulterous and blood is on their hands.

Ezekiel 23:45 (NIV)
But righteous men will sentence them to the punishment of women who commit adultery and shed blood, because they are adulterous and blood is on their hands.

Ezekiel 43:7 (NIV)
He said: "Son of man, this is the place of my throne and the place for the soles of my feet. This is where I will live among the Israelites forever. The house of Israel will never again defile my holy name--neither they nor their kings--by their prostitution and the lifeless idols of their kings at their high places.

Ezekiel 43:9 (NIV)
Now let them put away from me their prostitution and the lifeless idols of their kings, and I will live among them forever.

Hosea 1:2 (NIV)
When the LORD began to speak through Hosea, the LORD said to him, "Go, take to yourself an adulterous wife and children of unfaithfulness, because the land is guilty of the vilest adultery in departing from the LORD."

Hosea 2:2 (NIV)
Rebuke your mother, rebuke her, for she is not my wife, and I am not her husband. Let her remove the adulterous look from her face and the unfaithfulness from between her breasts.

Hosea 2:4 (NIV)
I will not show my love to her children, because they are the children of adultery.

Hosea 3:1 (NIV)
The LORD said to me, "Go, show your love to your wife again, though she is loved by another and is an adulteress. Love her as the LORD loves the Israelites, though they turn to other gods and love the sacred raisin cakes."

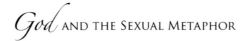

Hosea 3:3 (NIV)
Then I told her, "You are to live with me many days; you must not be a prostitute or be intimate with any man, and I will live with you."

Hosea 4:2 (NIV)
There is only cursing, lying and murder, stealing and adultery; they break all bounds, and bloodshed follows bloodshed.

Hosea 4:10 (NIV)
They will eat but not have enough; they will engage in prostitution but not increase, because they have deserted the LORD to give themselves to prostitution,

Hosea 4:12-15 (NIV)
They consult a wooden idol and are answered by a stick of wood. A spirit of prostitution leads them astray; they are unfaithful to their God. They sacrifice on the mountaintops and burn offerings on the hills, under oak, poplar and terebinth, where the shade is pleasant. Therefore your daughters turn to prostitution and your daughters-in-law to adultery. I will not punish your daughters when they turn to prostitution, nor your daughters-in-law when they commit adultery, because the men themselves consort with harlots and sacrifice with shrine prostitutes-- a people without understanding will come to ruin! Though you commit adultery, O Israel, let not Judah become guilty. "Do not go to Gilgal; do not go up to Beth Aven. And do not swear, 'As surely as the LORD lives!

Hosea 4:18 (NIV)
Even when their drinks are gone, they continue their prostitution; their rulers dearly love shameful ways.

Hosea 5:3-4 (NIV)
I know all about Ephraim; Israel is not hidden from me. Ephraim, you have now turned to prostitution; Israel is corrupt. Their deeds do not permit them to return to their God. A spirit of prostitution is in their heart; they do not acknowledge the LORD.

Hosea 6:10 (NIV)
I have seen a horrible thing in the house of Israel. There Ephraim is given to prostitution and Israel is defiled.

Hosea 9:1 (NIV)
Do not rejoice, O Israel; do not be jubilant like the other nations. For you have been unfaithful to your God; you love the wages of a prostitute at every threshing floor.

Joel 3:3 (NIV)
They cast lots for my people and traded boys for prostitutes; they sold girls for wine that they might drink.

Amos 7:17 (NIV)
Therefore this is what the LORD says: "'Your wife will become a prostitute in the city, and your sons and daughters will fall by the sword. Your land will be measured and divided up, and you yourself will die in a pagan country. And Israel will certainly go into exile, away from their native land.'"

Micah 1:7 (NIV)
All her idols will be broken to pieces; all her temple gifts will be burned with fire; I will destroy all her images. Since she gathered her gifts from the wages of prostitutes, as the wages of prostitutes they will again be used.

Nahum 3:4 (NIV)
All because of the wanton lust of a harlot, alluring, the mistress of sorceries, who enslaved nations by her prostitution and peoples by her witchcraft.

Matthew 5:27-28 (NIV)
You have heard that it was said, "Do not commit adultery." But I tell you that anyone who looks at a woman lustfully has already committed adultery with her in his heart.

Matthew 5:32 (NIV)
But I tell you that anyone who divorces his wife, except for marital unfaithfulness, causes her to become an adulteress, and anyone who marries the divorced woman commits adultery.

Matthew 12:39 (NIV)
He answered, "A wicked and adulterous generation asks for a miraculous sign! But none will be given it except the sign of the prophet Jonah.

Matthew 15:19 (NIV)
For out of the heart come evil thoughts, murder, adultery, sexual immorality, theft, false testimony, slander.

Matthew 16:4 (NIV)
A wicked and adulterous generation looks for a miraculous sign, but none will be given it except the sign of Jonah." Jesus then left them and went away.

Matthew 19:9 (NIV)
I tell you that anyone who divorces his wife, except for marital
unfaithfulness, and marries another woman commits adultery."

Matthew 19:18 (NIV)
"Which ones?" the man inquired. Jesus replied, "'Do not murder, do not
commit adultery, do not steal, do not give false testimony."

Matthew 21:31 (NIV)
"Which of the two did what his father wanted?" "The first," they answered.
Jesus said to them, "I tell you the truth, the tax collectors and the prostitutes
are entering the kingdom of God ahead of you."

Matthew 21:32 (NIV)
For John came to you to show you the way of righteousness, and you did
not believe him, but the tax collectors and the prostitutes did. And even after
you saw this, you did not repent and believe him.

Mark 7:21 (NIV)
[21] For from within, out of men's hearts, come evil thoughts, sexual
immorality, theft, murder, adultery,

Mark 8:38 (NIV)
If anyone is ashamed of me and my words in this adulterous and sinful
generation, the Son of Man will be ashamed of him when he comes in his
Father's glory with the holy angels."

Mark 10:11 (NIV)
He answered, "Anyone who divorces his wife and marries another woman
commits adultery against her.

Mark 10:12 (NIV)
And if she divorces her husband and marries another man, she commits
adultery.

Mark 10:19 (NIV)
"You know the commandments: 'Do not murder, do not commit adultery, do
not steal, do not give false testimony, do not defraud, honor your father and
mother.'"

Luke 15:30 (NIV)
But when this son of yours who has squandered your property with
prostitutes comes home, you kill the fattened calf for him!'

Luke 16:18 (NIV)
Anyone who divorces his wife and marries another woman commits adultery, and the man who marries a divorced woman commits adultery.

Luke 18:20 (NIV)
You know the commandments: 'Do not commit adultery, do not murder, do not steal, do not give false testimony, honor your father and mother.'"

John 8:3-4 (NIV)
The teachers of the law and the Pharisees brought in a woman caught in adultery. They made her stand before the group and said to Jesus, "Teacher, this woman was caught in the act of adultery."

Romans 2:22 (NIV)
You who say that people should not commit adultery, do you commit adultery? You who abhor idols, do you rob temples?

Romans 7:3 (NIV)
So then, if she marries another man while her husband is still alive, she is called an adulteress. But if her husband dies, she is released from that law and is not an adulteress, even though she marries another man.

Romans 13:9 (NIV)
The commandments, "Do not commit adultery," "Do not murder," "Do not steal," "Do not covet," and whatever other commandment there may be, are summed up in this one rule: "Love your neighbor as yourself."

1 Corinthians 6:9 (NIV)
Do you not know that the wicked will not inherit the kingdom of God? Do not be deceived: Neither the sexually immoral nor idolaters nor adulterers nor male prostitutes nor homosexual offenders

1 Corinthians 6:15-16 (NIV)
Do you not know that your bodies are members of Christ himself? Shall I then take the members of Christ and unite them with a prostitute? Never! Do you not know that he who unites himself with a prostitute is one with her in body? For it is said, "The two will become one flesh."

Hebrews 11:31 (NIV)
By faith the prostitute Rahab, because she welcomed the spies, was not killed with those who were disobedient.

James 2:11 (NIV)
For he who said, "Do not commit adultery," also said, "Do not murder."

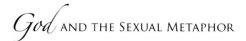

If you do not commit adultery but do commit murder, you have become a lawbreaker.

James 2:25 (NIV)
In the same way, was not even Rahab the prostitute considered righteous for what she did when she gave lodging to the spies and sent them off in a different direction?

James 4:4 (NIV)
You adulterous people, don't you know that friendship with the world is hatred toward God? Anyone who chooses to be a friend of the world becomes an enemy of God.

2 Peter 2:14 (NIV)
With eyes full of adultery, they never stop sinning; they seduce the unstable; they are experts in greed--an accursed brood!

Revelation 2:22 (NIV)
So I will cast her on a bed of suffering, and I will make those who commit adultery with her suffer intensely, unless they repent of her ways.

Revelation 14:8 (NIV)
A second angel followed and said, "Fallen! Fallen is Babylon the Great, which made all the nations drink the maddening wine of her adulteries."

Revelation 17:1-2 (NIV)
One of the seven angels who had the seven bowls came and said to me, "Come, I will show you the punishment of the great prostitute, who sits on many waters. With her the kings of the earth committed adultery and the inhabitants of the earth were intoxicated with the wine of her adulteries."

Revelation 17:4-5 (NIV)
The woman was dressed in purple and scarlet, and was glittering with gold, precious stones and pearls. She held a golden cup in her hand, filled with abominable things and the filth of her adulteries. [5] This title was written on her forehead: MYSTERY BABYLON THE GREAT THE MOTHER OF PROSTITUTES AND OF THE ABOMINATIONS OF THE EARTH.

Revelation 17:15-16 (NIV)
Then the angel said to me, "The waters you saw, where the prostitute sits, are peoples, multitudes, nations and languages. The beast and the ten horns you saw will hate the prostitute. They will bring her to ruin and leave her naked; they will eat her flesh and burn her with fire.

Revelation 18:3 (NIV)
For all the nations have drunk the maddening wine of her adulteries. The kings of the earth committed adultery with her, and the merchants of the earth grew rich from her excessive luxuries."

Revelation 18:9 (NIV)
When the kings of the earth who committed adultery with her and shared her luxury see the smoke of her burning, they will weep and mourn over her.

Revelation 19:2 (NIV)
For true and just are his judgments. He has condemned the great prostitute who corrupted the earth by her adulteries. He has avenged on her the blood of his servants.

GOD AND THE SEXUAL METAPHOR

ISBN 978-1-935434-77-1

Order books from www.gea-books.com/bookstore/
amazon.com; barnesandnoble.com
or any place good books are sold.

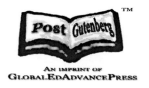

Post Gutenberg™

AN IMPRINT OF
GLOBAL ED ADVANCE PRESS